CHRONIC
PAIN
Management

T0178806

Thanthullu Vasu
Shyam Balasubramanian
Mahesh Kodivalasa
Pradeep Mukund Ingle

tfm Publishing Limited, Castle Hill Barns, Harley, Shrewsbury, SY5 6LX, UK
Tel: +44 (0)1952 510061; Fax: +44 (0)1952 510192
E-mail: info@tfmpublishing.com; Web site: www.tfmpublishing.com

Editing, design & typesetting: Nikki Bramhill BSc Hons Dip Law
Cover photo: © iStock.com
Butterfly vector sign
Credit: serkorkin; stock illustration ID: 510236902

First edition: © 2021
Paperback   ISBN: 978-1-910079-91-1
E-book editions: © 2021
ePub   ISBN: 978-1-910079-92-8
Mobi   ISBN: 978-1-910079-93-5
Web pdf   ISBN: 978-1-910079-94-2

Printed by Gutenberg Press Ltd., Gudja Road, Tarxien, GXQ 2902, Malta
Tel: +356 2398 2201; Fax: +356 2398 2290
E-mail: info@gutenberg.com.mt; Web site: www.gutenberg.com.mt

Contents

Foreword

"Divine is the task to relieve pain."
Hippocrates

Chronic pain affects a significant amount of the population. All healthcare professionals and clinicians need to have a basic knowledge of chronic pain. Even simple interventions can make a huge change in these suffering patients by improving their quality of life.

We realised that there is a scarcity of simple chronic pain books that could be used for day-to-day practice in our clinical life. Huge encyclopaedic textbooks might not serve the needs of exam-preparing candidates. This book covers the basics of chronic pain management that will be useful for all healthcare professionals in their clinical practise. Our aim is for topics to be relevant to multidisciplinary pain clinicians, general practitioners, anaesthetists, intensive care professionals, surgical and nursing staff, physiotherapists, psychologists, operating department professionals, healthcare managers and researchers who need a simple overview of the key topics in this subject. In addition, medical students and junior doctors will find this book very helpful to deal with their complex pain patients.

We are sure that this book will be an important tool in preparing for professional exams. Candidates preparing for the following examinations will find this book useful: the Royal College of Anaesthetists, London (FRCA), the Faculty of Pain Medicine, London (FFPMRCA), The College of

Anaesthesiologists of Ireland (FCAI), the European Society of Anaesthesiology (EDAIC), the European Society of Intensive Care Medicine (EDIC), the Australian and New Zealand College of Anaesthetists (FANZCA), the World Institute of Pain (FIPP/CIPS), the National Board of Examinations of India (Dip NB), and the American and Canadian Board examinations, as well as other competitive exams across the world.

We would like to thank Nikki Bramhill from tfm publishing, who has been an enormous motivation and support since we started with this idea. All our innovative ideas and dreams have been made possible only with the unrestricted help and support from Nikki and her team at tfm publishing.

We would also like to thank all the clinicians, healthcare professionals and trainees in the field of pain medicine, who have constantly encouraged our teaching and training courses, and given their constructive feedback. We thank them for their quest for knowledge with the aim of helping patients with chronic pain.

Finally, we thank you all for purchasing this book and encouraging us in our publishing endeavours. We wish you all the best for your future.

Dr Thanthullu Vasu MBBS MD DNB FRCA FFPMRCA Dip Pain Mgt
Consultant in Pain Medicine
University Hospitals of Leicester NHS Trust, UK

Dr Shyam Sundar Balasubramanian MBBS MD MSc FRCA FFPMRCA
Consultant in Anaesthetics and Pain Medicine
University Hospitals Coventry and Warwickshire NHS Trust, UK

Dr Mahesh Kodivalasa MBBS MD FRCA FFPMRCA
Consultant in Anaesthetics and Pain Medicine
University Hospitals of Leicester NHS Trust, UK

Dr Pradeep Mukund Ingle MBBS MD Dip Critical Care FRCA FFPMRCA
Consultant in Anaesthetics and Pain Medicine
University Hospitals of North Midlands, UK

Contributors

The Editors/Authors

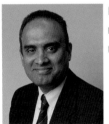

Dr Thanthullu Vasu
MBBS MD DNB FRCA
FFPMRCA Dip Pain Mgt

Consultant in Pain Medicine
University Hospitals of Leicester
NHS Trust, UK

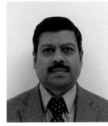

Dr Shyam Sundar Balasubramanian
MBBS MD MSc FRCA FFPMRCA

Consultant in Anaesthetics and Pain Medicine
University Hospitals Coventry and Warwickshire
NHS Trust, UK

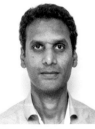

Dr Mahesh Kodivalasa
MBBS MD FRCA FFPMRCA

Consultant in Anaesthetics and Pain Medicine
University Hospitals of Leicester
NHS Trust, UK

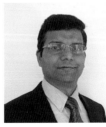

Dr Pradeep Mukund Ingle MBBS MD Dip Critical Care FRCA FFPMRCA

Consultant in Anaesthetics and Pain Medicine
University Hospitals of North Midlands, UK

Contributors

Dr Gopi Boora MBBS DFSRH
General Practitioner and Clinical Commissioning Group Governing Body
Member and Locality Chair, Leicester, UK

Dr Uday Idukallu MBBS MRCGP DGM DRCOG DFSRH PGCME
General Practitioner, Rotherham, UK

Dr Arul James MBBS MD FRCA
Advanced Pain Trainee, East Midlands Anaesthetic Training Rotation,
Leicester, UK

Dr Harnarine Murally MBBS FRCA MSc
Consultant in Anaesthetics and Pain Medicine, University Hospitals of North
Midlands NHS Trust, UK

Dr Ravindra Pochiraju MBBS MD EDIC FFICM
Specialty Doctor, University Hospitals of Leicester NHS Trust, Leicester, UK

Dr Ashok Puttappa MD FCAI AFRCA DiFPMCAI EDPM MSc DESRA
Consultant in Anaesthetics and Pain Medicine, University Hospitals of North
Midlands NHS Trust, UK

Dr Vanja Srbljak MD EDAIC FCAI EDRA FFPMRCA
Consultant in Anaesthetics and Pain Medicine, University Hospital of North
Midlands NHS Trust, UK

Dr Rajinikanth Sundara Rajan MD DA FRCA EDRA FFPMRCA
Consultant in Anaesthetics and Pain Medicine, University Hospitals of North
Midlands NHS Trust, UK

Abbreviations

°C	Degree Celsius
%	Percentage
5HT	5-hydroxy tryptamine or serotonin
A1	Analgesia first approach
AAGBI	Association of Anaesthetists of Great Britain and Ireland
ACE	Angiotensin-converting enzyme
ACR	American College of Rheumatology
ACT	Acceptance and commitment therapy
ACTH	Adrenocorticotrophic hormone
ADHD	Attention deficit hyperactivity disorder
AF	Atrial fibrillation
AKI	Acute kidney injury
ALARA	As low as reasonably achievable
AM	Amplitude modulation
AMPA	Alpha-amino 3-hydoxy-5-methyl-4-isoxazolepropionic acid
ARS	Acute radiation syndrome
ATP	Adenosine triphosphate
BD	*Bis die sumendum*, twice daily
BMI	Body Mass Index
BPI	Brief Pain Inventory
BPS	British Pain Society
Ca^{2+}	Calcium ions
cAMP	Cyclic adenosine monophosphate
CAPA tool	Clinically Aligned Pain Assessment tool
CBT	Cognitive behavioural therapy
cGMP	Cyclic guanosine monophosphate
CGRP	Calcitonin gene-related peptide

CKD	Chronic kidney disease
CNMP	Chronic non-malignant pain
CNS	Central nervous system
CO_2	Carbon dioxide
COVID	Coronavirus disease
COX	Cyclo-oxygenase
CPAQ	Chronic Pain Acceptance Questionnaire
CPCI	Chronic Pain Coping Inventory
CPOT	Critical care Pain Observation Tool
CPSP	Chronic post-surgical pain
CRIES scale	Crying, Requirement for oxygen, Increased vital signs, Grimacing, Sleeplessness scale
CRP	C-reactive protein
CRPS	Complex regional pain syndrome
CSF	Cerebrospinal fluid
CT scan	Computerised tomographic scan
CVS	Cardiovascular system
D_T	Absorbed dose
DEXA scan	Dual-energy X-ray absorptiometry scan
DMARDs	Disease-modifying antirheumatic drugs
DN4	Douleur Neuropathique 4 questionnaire
DNA	Deoxyribonucleic acid
DOAC	Direct oral anticoagulant
ECG	Electrocardiogram
eGFR	Estimated glomerular filtration rate
EMG	Electromyography
EMLA	Eutectic mixture of local anaesthetics
EQ-5D	EuroQoL score for Quality Assessment in five dimensions
ESR	Erythrocyte sedimentaion rate
EULAR	European League Against Rheumatism
eV	Electronvolt
FABER test	Flexion abduction external rotation test
FDA	U.S. Food and Drug Administration agency
FLACC scale	Face, Legs, Activity, Cry, Consolability scale
g	Gram
G protein	Guanine nucleotide-binding protein
GABA	Gamma aminobutyric acid
GAD	Generalised anxiety disorder

GET	Graded exercise therapy
GI	Gastrointestinal
Gy	Gray
H^+	Hydrogen ions
HADS	Hospital Anxiety and Depression Scale
Hb	Haemoglobin
HCPC	Health and Care Professionals Council
HLA	Human leucocyte antigen
HPA axis	Hypothalamopituitary adrenal axis
H_T	Equivalent dose
HTN	Hypertension
IAPT	Improving access to psychological therapies
IASP	International Association for the Study of Pain
ICD	International Classification of Diseases
ICHD	International Classification of Headache Disorders
IDDM	Insulin-dependent diabetes mellitus
IHD	Ischaemic heart disease
IL	Interleukin
IM	Intramuscular
IRMER	Ionising Radiation (Medical Exposure) Regulations
ITDD	Intrathecal drug delivery system
ITS	Iontophoretic transdermal system
IUGR	Intra-uterine growth retardation
IV	Intravenous
K^+	Potassium ions
keV	Kiloelectronvolt
kg	Kilogram
L	Litre
LA	Local anaesthetics
LANSS	Leeds Assessment of Neuropathic Symptoms and Signs questionnaire
LET	Linear energy transfer
LT	Leukotriene
MAOI	Monoamine oxidase inhibitor
ME	Myalgic encephalomyelitis
mg	Milligram
MGPQ	McGill Pain Questionnaire
MHRA	Medicines and Healthcare products Regulatory Agency

MHz	Mega Hertz
ml	Millilitre
mm	Millimetre
MRI scan	Magnetic resonance imaging scan
MRSA	Methicillin-resistant *Staphylococcus aureus*
mSv	MilliSievert
Na$^+$	Sodium ions
NAPQI	N-acetyl-p-benzoquinone imine
NCS	Nerve conduction studies
NHS	National Health Service
NICE	National Institute for Health and Care Excellence
NMDA	N-methyl-D-aspartate
NNH	Numbers needed to harm
NNT	Numbers needed to treat
NO	Nitric oxide
NSAID	Non-steroidal anti-inflammatory drug
O$_2$	Oxygen
OD	*Omne in die*, once daily
OTC	Over the counter
PA	Posteroanterior view
PABA	Para-aminobenzoic acid
PAG	Periaqueductal gray
PAINAD	Pain Assessment in Advanced Dementia scale
PASS	Pain Anxiety Symptoms Scale
PCA	Patient-controlled analgesia
PCS	Pain Catastrophising Scale
PDN	Painful diabetic neuropathy
PET	Positron emission tomography
PGE1	Prostaglandin E1
PGE2	Prostaglandin E2
PGI2	Prostaglandin I2 or prostacyclin
PHE	Public Health England
PHN	Post-herpetic neuralgia
PMP	Pain managment programme
PO	Per oral
PR	Per rectal
qds	*Quater die sumendum*, four times a day
QOL	Quality of life

QST	Quantitative sensory testing
RBC	Red blood cell
RF	Radiofrequency
RMP	Resting membrane potential
RVM	Rostral ventromedial medulla
SCS	Spinal cord stimulator
SD	Standard deviation
SI joint	Sacroiliac joint
SIGN	Scottish Intercollegiate Guidelines Network
SOCRATES	Site, Occurence, Character, Radiation, Associations, Time/ duration, Exacerbating/relieving factors, Severity (an acronym to assess pain)
SOPA	Survey of Pain Attitudes
SNRI	Serotonin norepinephrine reuptake inhibitor
SS scale	Symptom Severity scale
SSRI	Selective serotonin reuptake inhibitor
Sv	Sievert
TAP block	Transversus abdominis plane block
TCA	Tricyclic antidepressant
tds	*Ter die sumendus*, three times a day
TENS	Transcutaneous electrical nerve stimulation machine/ therapy
TIA	Transient ischaemic attack
TN	Trigeminal neuralgia
TNF-alpha	Tumour necrosis factor alpha
TP	Threshold potential
TRP-1	Tyrosinase-related protein 1
TUNAFISH	Mnemonic used to identify red flags (Trauma, Unexplained weight loss, Neurological, Age, Fever, Immunity, Steroid, History)
TXA_2	Thromboxane A2
UK	United Kingdom
VAS	Visual Analogue Scale
VIP	Vasoactive intestinal peptide
WDR neurons	Wide dynamic range neurons
WHO	World Health Organization
WPI	Widespread Pain Index
W_R	Weighting factor

Chapter 1

Pain — definition and classification

Shyam Balasubramanian

Pain is defined as "an unpleasant sensory and emotional experience associated with, or resembling that associated with, actual or potential tissue damage." The International Association for the Study of Pain (IASP) has recently revised this definition (2020).

Pain can be acute or chronic (■ Table 1.1). Chronic pain is defined as pain that lasts or recurs for longer than 3 months.

Table 1.1. Differences between acute and chronic pain.

Acute pain	Chronic pain
The normal, predicted physiological response to an adverse chemical, thermal or mechanical stimulus associated with surgery, trauma and acute illness.	A pain state which is persistent and in which the cause of the pain may not be apparent.
	May be associated with a long-term incurable or intractable medical condition or disease.
Time-limited.	
Responsive to therapy.	Difficult to treat.

Chronic pain can be classified in different ways. Mainly, it can be due to malignancy or chronic non-cancer pain. The term 'functional pain' is used when patients present with pain of no obvious organic origin. One simple classification for chronic non-cancer pain is shown in ■ Figure 1.1.

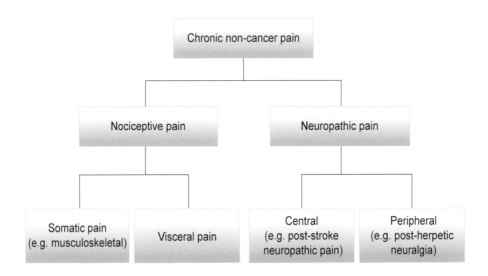

Figure 1.1. A simple classification for chronic non-cancer pain.

Recently, the IASP has developed a new classification system for chronic pain. Basically, this system divides chronic pain into two classes — chronic primary pain or chronic secondary pain.

Chronic primary pain

Chronic primary pain is defined as pain in one or more anatomical regions that:

- Persists or recurs for longer than 3 months.

- Is associated with significant emotional distress (e.g. anxiety, anger, frustration or depressed mood) and/or significant functional disability (interference in activities of daily life and participation in social roles).
- The symptoms are not better accounted for by another diagnosis.

The subclassification of chronic primary pain is as follows:

- Chronic widespread pain.
- Complex regional pain syndrome (CRPS).
- Chronic primary headache or orofacial pain.
- Chronic primary visceral pain.
- Chronic primary musculoskeletal pain.

Chronic secondary pain

Chronic secondary pain syndromes are linked to other diseases as the underlying cause, for which pain may initially be regarded as a symptom.

The subclassification of chronic secondary pain includes:

- Chronic cancer-related pain — pain caused by the cancer itself (by the primary tumour or by metastases) or by its treatment (surgery, chemotherapy and radiotherapy).
- Chronic post-surgical or post-traumatic pain — chronic pain that develops or increases in intensity after a surgical procedure or a tissue injury and persists beyond the healing process, i.e. at least 3 months after the surgery or tissue trauma.
- Chronic neuropathic pain — pain caused by a lesion or disease of the somatosensory nervous system.
- Chronic secondary headache or orofacial pain.
- Chronic secondary visceral pain — persistent or recurrent pain originating from internal organs of the head or neck region or of the thoracic, abdominal and pelvic cavities. It is often associated with emotional, cognitive and behavioural disability.
- Chronic secondary musculoskeletal pain — chronic pain in bones, joints and tendons arising from an underlying disease. It can be due

to persistent inflammation, associated with structural changes or caused by altered biomechanical function due to diseases of the nervous system.

In clinical practice, often these subclassifications coexist. For example, CRPS can present with a predominant neuropathic pain quality. Musculoskeletal back pain can cause sciatic nerve root irritation resulting in neuropathic radicular pain (sciatica). A Pancoast tumour (malignancy in the apex of the lung) can cause cancer pain, neuropathic pain due to involvement of the intercostal nerves and brachial plexus, musculoskeletal pain due to invasion into the intercostal muscles and chest wall, chemotherapy-induced peripheral neuropathic pain, etc.

Key Points

- Pain is an unpleasant sensory and emotional experience associated with, or resembling that associated with, actual or potential tissue damage.
- Pain can be acute or chronic; chronic pain can be primary or secondary.
- Often, various subclassifications of pain can coexist.

References

1. IASP terminology. The International Association for the Study of Pain. https://www.iasp-pain.org/Education/Content.aspx?ItemNumber=1698. Accessed on 20th July 2020.

2. Comment for IASP. https://www.iasp-pain.org/PublicationsNews/NewsDetail.aspx?ItemNumber=9218. Accessed on 20th July 2020.

3. Treede RD, Rief W, Barke A, *et al.* Chronic pain as a symptom or a disease: the IASP classification of chronic pain for the international classification of diseases: (ICD-11). *Pain* 2019; 160(1): 19-27.

Chapter 2

Assessing a patient with chronic pain

Pradeep Mukund Ingle

Challenges in pain assessment

The challenges in pain assessment are:

- There is no objective measure available currently.
- It is a sensory and emotional experience.
- The complex, multidimensional and subjective nature of pain makes assessment difficult.
- Pain presentation may be both physical and behavioural.
- The amount of pain does not always correlate with the amount of actual tissue damage.
- Tests such as a functional MRI or PET-brain activation may show the areas in the brain that 'light up' in response to pain but these are not practical to perform in each patient on a regular basis.

Why should we assess pain?

The management of pain is dependent upon its severity. The cause of pain can be ascertained through the process of pain assessment.

The three dimensions of pain (ABCs of pain)

- **A**ffective-motivational — relates to the emotional/suffering aspects in pain.

5

- Sensory-discriminative (**b**ehaviour) — sensory aspect of pain which is described in intensity, location and temporal (relates to time) aspects.
- **C**ognitive-evaluative — this relates to how pain is interpreted by the patient, and the resultant impact of pain on the patient's function and quality of life (QOL).

The structured assessment of pain

The structured assessment of pain is outlined in ■ Table 2.1.

Table 2.1. The structured assessment of pain.

- ■ History.
- ■ Examination and physical signs.
- ■ Investigations to determine the cause (or rule out the suspected causes).
- ■ Specialised tests if needed.
- ■ Pain scales — unidimensional and multidimensional scales, diagnostic pain questionnaire scales.
- ■ Pain scales in special populations, e.g. dementia, non-verbal adults, etc.

History

- The characteristics of pain (acronym — SOCRATES):
  - S — site of pain;
  - O — how did the pain start? What exactly was the patient doing when the pain started?
  - C — character of pain. What does it feel like? e.g. burning, tingling, shooting pain in the case of neuropathic pain vs. a sharp and localised nature in nociceptive pain;
  - R — radiation of pain. Where does the pain go from its original site?

- A — associated symptoms with pain, e.g. vomiting;
- T — time/duration of pain. To differentiate acute vs. chronic/persistent pain (>3 months);
- E — exacerbating and relieving factors, e.g. pain in trigeminal neuralgia is exacerbated/precipitated by sensory stimulation of the affected area over the face. Also, in spinal stenosis, extension of the spine worsens the pain and flexion of the spine can ease the pain;
- S — severity of the pain. Obtain a pain score.

- Impact on life on sleep, social and marital life. It is common for patients with chronic pain to have an adverse impact on sleep. Also, patients with poor sleep hygiene tend to report worse pain scores.
- Medical/surgical history. A medical history enables us to plan future management, and look for any challenges such as bipolar disorder, depression, various heart conditions, diabetes, etc., that can influence pain management. A surgical history can be helpful to understand the origin of the pain, for example, in chronic post-surgical pain.
- Red flags to rule out warning signs.
- Treatment history. It helps us to understand the effectiveness and side effects/complications of previous treatments from a pain point of view. It can also help in predicting the drug interactions based on the current medications and treatments patients are receiving.
- Psychology. This is more important in chronic pain states. The presence of pre-existing conditions such as anxiety and depression can exacerbate chronic pain conditions. Catastrophisation can aggravate pain conditions as well.
- Yellow flags. These are the factors that may indicate the potential for ongoing disability in patients with chronic pain.
- Psychosocial history. It is important to know about situations surrounding the patient, including family support, family members with painful conditions, compensation/litigation issues, work issues, etc. Various studies show that patients with family support often do better with chronic pain management than those without any support system. In addition, various factors such as smoking and a lack of work satisfaction are associated with back pain.
- Differentiate nociceptive vs. neuropathic pain. Listen to the verbal descriptors of the patient, e.g. neuropathic pain can have associated descriptors such as tingling, pins and needles, prickling, a crawling sensation, burning, stabbing, shooting, like an electrical shock, etc.

Examination

Generic points to be included in the examination are:

- Gait and walking aid requirement.
- Ability to sit and stand up.
- General mood.

A further site-specific examination includes:

- Inspection — colour changes, trophic changes, hair loss in painful area, scars.
- Range of movements — active and passive.
- Palpation — tenderness, swelling, signs of allodynia or hyperalgesia over the painful area.
- Neurological examination for back and neck pain.

Physical changes

- Physiological signs — increased heart rate, blood pressure, respiratory rate, nausea, pallor, sweating, pupil dilation, increased muscle tone are more important in acute pain.
- Using physiological measures in isolation will not result in a meaningful measure if a patient has a persistent pain condition.
- Physical signs — changes in temperature, colour, muscle wasting, muscle spasm can indicate the organic condition associated with chronic pain.
- Visual signs of pain including facial expressions and emotional changes should not be missed. Patients may not be necessarily able to communicate their pain and these signs can be useful in giving an indication of the severity of pain. Examples include: facial expression — decreased or increased eye contact, tears or grimacing; emotional changes — anger, sadness or a change in mood; a distanced patient — becoming quiet, withdrawn and uncommunicative during examination.

Specific tests

Specific tests should be used as indicated, e.g. a positive Carnett's sign can suggest likely abdominal wall pain and a negative sign suggests likely visceral pain; various provocative tests for sacroiliac (SI) joint pain like the FABER test, thigh thrust test and Gaenslen's test.

Special tests — quantitative sensory testing (QST)

QST systematically tests sensory and pain thresholds using specialised equipment which can help demonstrate nerve dysfunction. It is performed usually in specialised or research settings only. It allows the determination of pain and sensation thresholds by the non-invasive application of up to 12 different sensory stimuli of known intensity which are then compared with average sensory thresholds.

Various diagnostic investigations including structural imaging (MRI scans, CT scans), functional assessment (EMG/NCS) and histological assessment (nerve biopsies) may have to be undertaken to determine the cause and decide subsequent management.

Measurement of pain — pain scales

Various pain scales can be used to quantify pain. Given the complex nature of pain, it is sensible to classify these scales based on its utility.

Unidimensional pain scales

The patient assigns a value to the intensity and severity of pain. These are categorical rating scales:

- Visual analogue scale — unmarked scale with one end showing no pain and the other end showing severe pain. The patient places a mark on this scale to indicate pain severity.
- Numerical rating scale — rated and continuous scale from "0 to 10" or from "0 to 100" for quantifying pain.

- Verbal rating scale — non-continuous pain scale classifying pain from 0 to 4 with verbal descriptors like none, mild, moderate, severe and excruciating.
- Picture scales — useful in children, patients with poor language skills and those with a learning disability:
  - Wong-Baker FACES pain scale — categorical rating scale, consisting of a series of different facial expressions (ranging from "no hurt" to "worst hurt"). The patient is asked to point at the appropriate face that represents their pain dimensions. This is used in children more than 3 years of age;
  - Pieces of Hurt scale — useful for children aged 3-6 years old. The child is shown four pieces of the same item with each piece representing "how much it hurts". The child is asked how many "pieces does it hurt", to represent their pain. Any toy with four similar pieces (e.g. poker chips, pieces of toy pizza, etc.) can be used.

Multidimensional pain scales

These assess the severity of pain along with its impact on life by scoring the factors that impact the patient. They are usually used in the assessment of chronic pain conditions:

- Brief Pain Inventory — available in both long form and short form. It is scored as a mean of seven items of daily activities that are interfered with due to pain including general activity, walking, work, mood, enjoyment of life, relations with others and sleep.
- McGill Pain Questionnaire (MGPQ) — available in a short form MGPQ as well. It has four parts to assess pain: the first part relates to locating the pain sites; the second part to record the pain experience with time; the third part has 20 sets of pain verbal descriptors to select from; and the fourth part is to represent the intensity of pain.
- Clinically Aligned Pain Assessment (CAPA) Tool — for assessing acute pain. It scores five domains including comfort, change in pain, pain control, functioning and sleep.

Diagnostic pain questionnaires

These are used to differentiate neuropathic pain from nociceptive pain. These are complex questionnaires and are usually completed with a clinician's help:

- The Leeds Assessment of Neuropathic Symptoms and Signs (LANSS) — consists of seven questions which include five pain questions and two clinical sign questions. A score of 12 or more suggests neuropathic mechanisms are likely to be contributing to pain. This is commonly used in the UK.
- The Douleur Neuropathique 4 (DN4) — consists of a first part exploring the symptoms related to a patient's pain and a second part related to the examination of the painful part. A score of 4 or more indicates a likely probability of neuropathic pain.
- Pain DETECT — a screening questionnaire for determining a neuropathic pain component (initially designed for patients with low back pain). A cut-off value of 13 or more indicates a neuropathic component for the pain.

Other pain scales for specialised groups

Children

- FLACC scale — Face, Legs, Activity, Cry, Consolability scale with each point given 0 to 2 as scores. Scores of 1-3 indicate mild discomfort, scores of 4-6 indicate moderate pain and scores of 7-10 indicate severe pain. This is useful for children (2 to 8 years old) and older non-verbal children/adults.
- Revised FLACC scale — designed for cognitively impaired children.
- CRIES scale — validated from 32 weeks of gestational age to 6 months. It includes five categories scored from 0 to 2, namely Crying, Requirement for oxygen to maintain saturation above 95%, Increased vital signs (blood pressure and heart rate), Grimacing and Sleeplessness.

Dementia patients

- ABBEY Pain scale — a behavioural pain assessment tool that grades the measures of distress to give a pain score. This is useful in cognitively impaired patients. It is more commonly used in the UK. Scores of less than 2 indicate no pain, 3-7 indicate mild pain, 8-13 indicate moderate pain and 14 or more indicate severe pain.
- PAINAD — Pain Assessment in Advanced Dementia scale — uses five domains of discomfort behaviour with a score from 0 to 2 each, giving a maximum score of 10.

Non-verbal patients

- COMFORT scale — for non-verbal patients including children, cognitively impaired adults or sedated patients in the ICU. It uses seven domains to assess pain, namely, Alertness, Calmness, Respiratory distress, Crying, Physical movement, Muscle tone and Facial tension.

Key Points

- Appropriate pain assessment is the key to management of both acute and chronic pain.
- Structured pain assessment requires a careful history, examination, assessing physical signs, performing specialised tests and investigations as needed.
- Red and yellow flags need careful evaluation for optimising immediate management and addressing psychosocial issues, respectively.

References

1. Jackson MA, Simpson KH. Chronic back pain. *Contin Educ Anaesth Crit Care Pain* 2006; 6(4): 152-5.

2. E-learning for health — E-Pain.

3. Bendinger T, Plunkett N. Measurement in pain medicine. *BJA Educ* 2016; 16(9): 310-5.

4. Abe H, Sumitani M, Matsubayashi Y, *et al*. Validation of pain severity assessment using the PainDETECT questionnaire. *Int J Anesth Pain Med* 2017; 3(1): 3.

Chapter 3

Physiology of chronic pain

Mahesh Kodivalasa

Nociception is the neural mechanism by which an individual detects the presence of a potentially tissue-harming stimulus.

Nociceptors

- IASP definition — "high-threshold sensory receptors of the peripheral somatosensory system capable of encoding and transducing painful stimuli."
- Nociceptors are the free nerve endings of primary afferent Aδ and C fibres with their cell bodies located in the dorsal root ganglion.
- Nociceptors are ubiquitous in distribution and stimulated by mechanical, thermal or chemical stimuli.
- Three main types are described:
  - mechanoreceptors;
  - silent nociceptors;
  - polymodal mechano-heat nociceptors.

Primary afferent fibres (first-order afferents)

- Aδ and C fibres carry noxious sensory information.
- Aδ fibres respond to mechanical and thermal stimuli.
- C fibres (are polymodal) respond to mechanical, chemical and thermal stimuli.
- Aδ and C fibres synapse with second-order afferent neurons in the dorsal horn of the spinal cord.

- Primary afferent terminals release a number of excitatory neurotransmitters.

Dorsal horn of the spinal cord

- Aδ fibres synapse predominantly in Rexed laminas I and V, while C fibres synapse predominantly in laminas I, II and V.
- Second-order neurons are either nociceptive-specific or wide dynamic range (WDR) neurons.
- Nociceptive-specific neurons (located predominantly in laminas I and II) serve only noxious stimuli.
- WDR neurons (in lamina V) receive both non-noxious and noxious input from Aβ, Aδ and C fibres.
- Complex interactions occur in the dorsal horn.

Ascending tracts in the spinal cord (second-order afferent fibres)

- There are mainly two ascending pain pathways: the spinothalamic and spinoreticular tracts.

Spinothalamic tract

- The axons of second-order neurons cross to the contralateral side of the spinal cord and end in the thalamus, reticular formation, nucleus raphe magnus and the periaqueductal gray.
- The lateral (neo) spinothalamic tract projects mainly on to the ventral posterolateral nucleus of the thalamus and carries discriminative aspects of pain (location, intensity and duration).
- The medial (paleo) spinothalamic tract projects on to the medial thalamus and is responsible for mediating the autonomic and unpleasant emotional components of pain.

Spinoreticular tract

- The fibres decussate to reach the brainstem reticular formation, before projecting on to the thalamus, hypothalamus and to the cortex.
- This pathway is involved in the emotional aspects of pain.

Third-order afferent fibres

- Thalamic projections relay information to the higher cortical centres (the pain matrix).

The pain matrix

- Although the somatosensory cortex is important for the localisation of pain, the large brain network (pain matrix) is activated.
- The pain matrix comprises the primary and secondary somatosensory cortex, insula, anterior cingulate cortex and prefrontal cortex.

The mechanism of nociception involves transduction, transmission and perception; in addition, signal modulation also plays an important role. This can be facilitatory upregulation or inhibitory downregulation.

Inhibitory modulation

Descending inhibition

- The periaqueductal gray (PAG) in the midbrain and the rostral ventromedial medulla (RVM) are two important areas involved in descending inhibitory modulation.
- Descending pathways project on to the dorsal horn and inhibit pain transmission.
- These pathways are monoaminergic, utilising noradrenaline and serotonin as neurotransmitters.

Inhibition at the dorsal horn level (gate control — ■ Figure 3.1)

- Tactile non-noxious stimuli are carried by Aβ fibres. The faster Aβ fibres synapse on to and activate inhibitory interneurons in the dorsal horn. These interneurons in turn project on to and inhibit pain signals transmitted via relatively slower Aδ and C fibres.
- Glycine and gamma aminobutyric acid (GABA) are the main inhibitory neurotransmitters.
- Spinal inhibitory interneurons also store and release endogenous opioids.
- TENS machine treatment is based on the gate control theory.

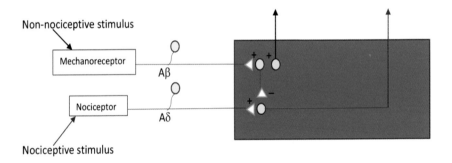

Figure 3.1. The gate control theory.

Facilitatory modulation

Peripheral sensitization

Primary hyperalgesia

- Inflammatory mediators (histamine, serotonin, bradykinin, prostaglandins, cytokines, H^+, K^+, etc.) are released from damaged tissue.

- These inflammatory mediators can stimulate nociceptors and reduce the activation threshold of nociceptors.
- Antidromic release of substance P from the afferent nerve endings also plays a role.

Secondary hyperalgesia (central mediated peripheral sensitization)

- IASP definition — "area of central mediated hyperalgesia that surrounds the area of initial injury."
- Involves histamine, serotonin, bradykinin, PGE2, leukotrienes, substance P, CGRP, etc., as neurochemical mediators.

Central sensitization

Central sensitization mainly involves two mechanisms:

- Wind-up and sensitization of second-order neurons.
- Receptive field expansion in the dorsal horn — by the recruitment of WDR neurons.

The main neurochemical mediators are: substance P, CGRP, VIP, cholecystokinin, angiotensin, glutamate, aspartate and inflammatory mediators (IL and TNF-α).

The main channels and receptors involved are: Na^+ channels, G-protein coupled receptors, TRP1 receptors, N-methyl-D-aspartate (NMDA) receptors, α-amino-3-hydroxy-5-methyl-4-isoxazolepropionic acid (AMPA) receptors and kainate receptors.

The final common pathway involves the production of NO, increased intracellular calcium, and phosphorylation of substrate proteins.

A knowledge of pain physiology helps in the understanding and development of various pharmacological and non-pharmacological approaches in the management of pain; for example, it is important to understand the role of anti-inflammatory agents, prostaglandin synthesis inhibitors, monoaminergic neurotransmitter upregulators, calcium channel blockers, NMDA antagonists, etc.

Key Points

- Nociception is the neural mechanism by which an individual detects the presence of a potentially tissue-harming noxious stimulus.
- Transduction, transmission, modulation and perception are the four main mechanisms involved. An imbalance in upregulatory and downregulatory pain modulation mechanisms is a key factor in chronic pain maintenance.
- The overall experience of pain is complex and subjective, affected by various factors such as genetics, emotions, cognition, mood, beliefs, past encounters, etc.

References

1. Scholz J. Mechanisms of chronic pain. *Mol Pain* 2014; 10(Suppl 1): O15.
2. Feizerfan A, Sheh G. Transition from acute to chronic pain. *Contin Educ Anaesth Crit Care Pain* 2015; 15(2): 98-102.

Chapter 4

The biopsychosocial model

Thanthullu Vasu

The biopsychosocial model helps us to understand and manage chronic pain in a better way by considering the pain and patient as a whole:

- Bio — how the physiology has been affected and the pathology/cause.
- Psycho — emotions and behaviours, causing persistence and associated beliefs.
- Social — how other circumstances have an effect, e.g. economical, environmental, cultural, work issues, etc.

When it was described by George Engel in 1977, the focus was to expand the biomedical model and consider the need to look at the body and the mind. It is well proven that pain, suffering and disability depend on a variety of cognitive and affective factors. Evaluation of pain needs reliance on the individual's perceptions.

While the previous decade focused on chronic pain clinicians looking more at psychological factors (e.g. coping skills, catastrophisation, etc.), recently, more focus has been given on social factors (e.g. family circumstances/relationships, economical situation, benefits system, etc.) in causing the persistence of chronic pain. Social outcomes can include a return-to-work success rate as well as resolution of legal issues or benefit claim issues.

These factors should be looked together as a continuum; this model helps to provide a multidimensional multimodal comprehensive treatment plan, individualised to the needs of the specific patient. Any pain clinic treatment should not only alter physical contributors, but also change the patient's behaviours, regardless of the patient's specific pathophysiology and without necessarily controlling pain as such.

The biopsychosocial model is commonly integrated into many pain management programmes and pain interventions. It helps patients to regain function and improve their quality of life.

Although many textbooks propose a Venn-diagram model for enclosing all three aspects, we have depicted these aspects in ■ Figures 4.1. and 4.2 — to express the fact that one facet can worsen the other significantly; this also reminds us of the most forgotten social aspect of chronic pain!

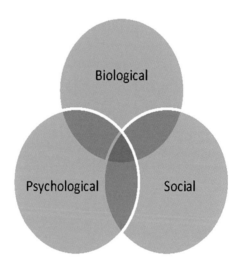

Figure 4.1. The biopsychosocial model.

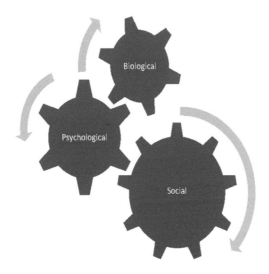

Figure 4.2. A complex interaction of biological, psychological and social factors.

Key Points

- The biopsychosocial model helps to manage chronic pain in a better way.
- Psychological factors and associated beliefs cause persistence of chronic pain.
- Social factors are usually forgotten and need to be evaluated for a better outcome.

References

1.   Engel G. The need for a new medical model: a challenge for biomedicine. *Science* 1977; 196: 129-36.

2.   Turk DC. Assess the person, not just the pain. *Pain Clinic Updates* 1993; 1(3): 1-3.

3.   IASP fact sheet no. 7. Evidence-based invasive treatment of chronic musculoskeletal pain. Global year against musculoskeletal pain 2009-2010. The International Association for the Study of Pain, 2017.

Chapter 5

Back pain

Shyam Balasubramanian

Most of the population will experience back pain at some time in their life. Mostly this is a self-limiting condition that settles with reassurance, simple analgesics, minimal rest and physical therapy. In a proportion of people with back pain, the symptoms persist and affect their quality of life. Chronic back pain remains one of the leading causes for clinical consultation, affecting employment and causing significant disability. The direct and indirect impact of back pain on healthcare costs and society is huge.

Classification

Patients presenting with back pain can be categorised into three groups:

- Simple mechanical back pain +/- referred pain to the lower limbs.
- Back pain + radicular pain (due to nerve root irritation — 'sciatica').
- Serious spinal pathology.

The term 'mechanical' refers to 'movement' and is generally due to a musculoskeletal cause. Not all pain radiating to the leg is 'sciatica'. In most patients with back and leg pain, this is due to a musculoskeletal cause with referred pain to the lower limbs. Mechanical back pain can originate from the bone, joints, discs or the adjacent soft tissues such as muscles and ligaments.

A smaller proportion have true nerve root irritation at the spinal level (due to disc protrusion, bony foraminal stenosis, etc.), resulting in neuropathic radicular pain (sciatica).

Serious spinal pathology is rare. However, the first step in the assessment of back pain is to eliminate 'red flags' secondary to serious spinal pathology. A mnemonic to identify the red flags is TUNA FISH:

- Trauma, history of a fall.
- Unexplained weight loss/history of malignancy.
- Neurological findings: cauda equina syndrome (unsteady gait, perineal numbness and sphincter disturbance).
- Age >55 years.
- Fever/systemic illness.
- Immunocompromised.
- Steroid use.
- History of HIV, tuberculosis, cancer.

Assessment

Assessment of a patient with back pain includes a history, an examination and investigations.

History

A mnemonic for eliciting a systematic pain history is SOCRATES:

- Site — lumbosacral, thoracic (uncommon, need to rule out red flags).
- Onset — insidious, trauma, repetitive sprain, lifting, twisting.
- Character — aching (musculoskeletal), paraesthesia, burning, electric shock, etc. (neuropathic).
- Radiation — to the lower limbs — referred? (musculoskeletal), radicular? (neuropathic).
- Associated symptoms — systemic upset? Abdominopelvic symptoms with referred pain to the back?
- Time/duration — how long? Intermittent? Constant? (With constant non-mechanical pain, there is a need to rule out red flags.)

- Exacerbating/relieving factors — musculoskeletal pain worsens with activity and is relieved by rest. Coughing, sneezing and bending forward may increase disc-related spinal pain.
- Severity — at rest, with movements.

Examination

Clinical methods alone can be less specific in the diagnosis of the precise cause for back pain. This is because of the complex inter-linked structural arrangement in the lumbosacral spine. A number of anatomical structures such as bone, joints, discs, and soft tissues can be the pain generators. To add to the complexity, patients with functional pain disorders can also present with back pain with no obvious structural cause to explain their symptoms.

Systematic examination may help to differentiate musculoskeletal back pain from back pain with nerve root irritation (radicular pain):

- Inspection — gait, conspicuous skeletal abnormalities (kyphosis, scoliosis), loss of lumbar lordosis, paraspinal muscle wasting (chronic disuse), assessing the range of movement around the lower back (forward flexion, backward extension, lateral flexion and rotation), heel (L5) — toe (S1) walking.
- Palpation — midline or paraspinal tenderness, muscle spasm, tenderness over any specific anatomical area such as the sacroiliac joint.
- Provocation tests — e.g. a straight leg raising test to identify any nerve root irritation.
- Neurological tests (if there are radicular features) — motor, sensory, reflexes. The common nerve roots involved are L4, L5 and S1 (■ Table 5.1).

Table 5.1. Tests for radicular features.

	L4	L5	S1
Sensory	Anterior thigh Inner aspect of the leg	Outer aspect of the leg Dorsum of the foot Great toe	Lateral border of the foot Sole
Motor	Quadriceps	Dorsiflexion of the ankle	Plantar flexion of the ankle
Reflex	Knee jerk	Ankle jerk	Ankle jerk

Investigations

Investigations have limitations in musculoskeletal low back pain. X-rays have limited value. MRI scans often show non-specific changes which can unnecessarily cause more concern.

Patients with serious spinal pathology, presenting with red flags, need an urgent MRI scan. Patients with radicular pain in the legs (due to nerve root irritation) may benefit from having an MRI scan. This is mainly to ascertain whether clinical findings correlate with the radiological findings, in particular, if a targeted injection therapy or a surgery is planned.

Management

Management of acute back pain

- Rule out red flags.
- Avoid over-investigation.
- Simple analgesics. Opioids for pain and muscle relaxants such as diazepam can be used only for a short period of time. The evidence for long-term use is sparse and can be counterproductive.

- Only brief periods of bed rest.
- Encourage early ambulation and return to a normal activity level.
- Physical therapy.

Management of chronic back pain

The management of chronic back pain is multimodal and multidisciplinary; a biopsychosocial approach. The objectives are symptom relief and functional restoration.

Apart from reassurance and encouragement to maintain a reasonable level of physical activity, the strategies include:

- Physical therapy.
- Pharmacotherapy.
- Injection therapy.
- Neuromodulation.
- Psychological interventions.
- Surgery.

These are not mutually exclusive treatment options — but are often provided in combination. Sometimes, a psychological component may play an important role in affecting the pain experience. Interventions such as cognitive behavioural therapy can be helpful in those patients.

Physical therapy

In chronic back pain management, regular physical exercise is recommended to avoid disability. Stretching and strengthening exercises, apart from improving general fitness, can be effective with back pain management. Adherence to regular home exercise is important to achieve long-term goals.

Pharmacotherapy

It is important to differentiate musculoskeletal back pain (+/- referred pain to the legs) from radicular pain (due to nerve root irritation), as the choice of medications for these conditions will be different.

With musculoskeletal pain, medications such as paracetamol, non-steroidal anti-inflammatories (ibuprofen, diclofenac, naproxen, etc.) can be useful.

With radicular pain (neuropathic pain), medications such as amitriptyline, gabapentin, pregabalin, duloxetine can be useful.

In either of these back-pain conditions, if opioids are considered — then the pros and cons need to be weighed up on an individual case basis. In a select group of patients, a steady non-incremental dose of opioids may be helpful for pain relief and facilitate functional restoration.

Injection therapy

When conservative measures provide suboptimal relief, minimally-invasive injection therapy may be offered for diagnostic and treatment purposes in the management of low back pain. Injections should be a component of a 'multimodal approach'.

Musculoskeletal back pain may respond to injection procedures such as muscle trigger point injections, facet joint nerve blocks (+/- radiofrequency denervation), sacroiliac joint injections, etc.

Radicular pain (due to nerve irritation) may respond to epidural injections (interlaminar lumbar epidural, caudal epidural, transforaminal epidural) and nerve root/dorsal root ganglion blocks, etc.

Neuromodulation

Spinal cord stimulation is a neuromodulation technique offered in selected centres for radicular pain unresponsive to conventional treatments.

Psychological interventions

Cognitive behavioural therapy (CBT), acceptance and commitment therapy (ACT), a mindfulness-based approach, and a pain management programme (PMP), etc., can be helpful.

Surgery

Lumbar decompression surgery for radicular pain; this should only be considered if the pain is not resolving after other treatments used for chronic back pain have been tried.

Barriers to recovery

There are some psychosocial barriers to recovery — commonly described as 'yellow flags'.

These include:

- A strong belief that activity-related pain is harmful.
- Low mood, negative attitude, social withdrawal.
- Dissatisfaction at work.
- Problems with litigation/claims/compensation.
- Sickness behaviour.
- Overprotective family.
- Lack of family support.

Key Points

- Back pain can be: (i) simple mechanical back pain; (ii) radicular pain (sciatica); or (iii) due to serious spinal pathology.
- Assessment includes a history, an examination and investigations.
- Recognising 'red flags' is important.
- Management is multimodal.
- The goal is symptom relief and functional rehabilitation.

References

1. Low back pain and sciatica in over 16s: assessment and management. NICE guideline, NG59. London: National Institute for Health and Care Excellence, 2016. https://www.nice.org.uk/guidance/ng59. Accessed on 6th July 2020.

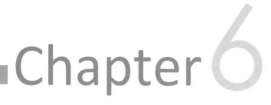

Chapter 6

Neck pain

Thanthullu Vasu

Neck pain is common and can affect 15% of the population at some point in their lives. It is more common in middle age and affects more women. Risk factors include high physical job demands, a history of low back or neck injury, low social support and smoking. Non-specific neck pain usually resolves within a few weeks.

Let us use the same pattern as our previous chapter to look at the history and examination. To remind us from the previous chapter, the mnemonic to identify the red flags is TUNA FISH:

- Trauma, history of a fall.
- Unexplained weight loss/history of malignancy.
- Neurological findings.
- Age >55 years.
- Fever/systemic illness.
- Immunocompromised.
- Steroid use.
- History of HIV, tuberculosis, cancer.

Assessment

Assessment of a patient with neck pain includes a history, an examination and investigations.

History

Let us use the same mnemonic for eliciting a systematic pain history as in the previous chapter — SOCRATES:

- Site — midline or paraspinal.
- Onset — insidious, trauma, repetitive sprain, lifting, with particular movement/whiplash.
- Character — pain or stiffness? Neuropathic features?
- Radiation — to the upper limbs — referred? (musculoskeletal), radicular? (neuropathic).
- Associated symptoms — systemic upset, dizziness, headache or radiating pain to the shoulder or upper limbs, visual or auditory symptoms, temporomandibular symptoms?
- Time/duration — how long? Intermittent? Constant? (With constant non-mechanical pain, there is a need to rule out red flags.)
- Exacerbating/relieving factors — musculoskeletal pain worsens with activity and is relieved by rest.
- Severity — at rest, with movements.

Examination

Clinical methods alone can be less specific in the diagnosis of the precise cause for the neck pain.

Table 6.1. The Quebec Task Force classification for whiplash injury.

Grade	
Grade 0	Asymptomatic, no signs; need reassurance/education.
Grade I	Pain, stiffness or tenderness, absent signs; need simple analgesics.
Grade II	Pain, stiffness or tenderness, with musculoskeletal signs (decreased range of movements, joint tenderness); need non-opioids or NSAIDs.
Grade III	As Grade II with neurological involvement (sensory deficits, motor weakness, absent reflexes); need radiography and opioids for a limited period if severe and acute.
Grade IV	As above with dislocation or fracture with or without spinal cord injury; need specialised imaging, medications and referral to a specialist surgeon.

The Quebec Task Force classification for whiplash injury defines whiplash as an acceleration-deceleration mechanism of energy transfer to the neck and is graded as Grade 0-IV (■ Table 6.1).

Investigations

An MRI scan can be useful for radicular pain or myelopathy or in severe injury; in other cases of simple mechanical pain, the value of this investigation is limited.

Management

The aim is to reduce symptoms and improve function/quality of life. Patient education and an explanation will help in the success of treatment. A multimodal approach using a biopsychosocial model is the key to recovery.

Physical therapy

Specific neck strengthening exercises have a moderate level of evidence.

Complementary therapies

TENS machines and acupuncture have been successfully used as part of a comprehensive plan in many pain clinics. Hot or cold packs might help in neck pain also.

Pharmacotherapy

In musculoskeletal neck pain, non-steroidal anti-inflammatory medications (ibuprofen, diclofenac, naproxen, etc.) can be used only for short-term use, if appropriate.

In radicular pain (neuropathic pain), medications such as amitriptyline, gabapentin, pregabalin or duloxetine can be useful and can be used as per the NICE guidelines (see Chapter 8, Neuropathic pain).

Injection therapy

When conservative measures provide suboptimal relief, minimally-invasive injection therapy may be offered for diagnostic and treatment purposes in the management of neck pain. Injections should be a component of a multimodal approach.

Musculoskeletal neck pain may respond to injection procedures such as muscle trigger point injections or a cervical medial branch block (+/- radiofrequency denervation), depending on the examination findings.

Psychological interventions

Cognitive behavioural therapy (CBT), acceptance and commitment therapy (ACT), mindfulness-based interventions and a pain management programme (PMP) have a role to play in chronic persistent neck pain.

Key Points

- Rule out any red flags; the patient may need investigations and an appropriate immediate referral.
- Education and reassurance are a vital part of the treatment plan.
- Conduct a history, an examination and assessment, and proceed to a comprehensive multidisciplinary multimodal management plan based on the biopsychosocial model.
- Opioids should be used only for short periods if needed; beware of issues related to opioids.

References

1.   IASP fact sheet no. 18. Neck pain. Global year against musculoskeletal pain, 2009-2010. The International Association for the Study of Pain, 2017.
2.   Tameem A, Kapur S, Mutagi H, *et al*. Whiplash injury. *Contin Educ Anaesth Crit Care Pain* 2014; 14(4): 167-70.

Chapter 7

Osteoarthritis and osteoporosis

Thanthullu Vasu

Osteoarthritis

Osteoarthritis is the most common joint disorder and is the commonest cause of pain and disability worldwide. Knee arthritis occurs in 37% of people over the age of 60 years. No proven treatment can stop the progression of osteoarthritis. It is more common in an obese individual and more common in women than men.

Aetiopathology

The pathophysiology includes a localised loss of cartilage, remodelling of adjacent bone and inflammation. There might be a slow and efficient repair process following the initial trauma, which if not compensated can cause symptoms. There is extreme variability between clinical features and the outcome.

Primary hypersensitization is due to localised inflammation; secondary hyperalgesia can follow due to central nervous system changes with enhanced sensitivity causing pain outside the area of injury. Psychological factors can play an important role in the response and outcome of the condition.

Assessment

For a diagnosis, the patient should have pain and any five of the following criteria:

- Age >50 years.
- Stiffness <30 minutes.
- Bony tenderness.
- Crepitus.
- Bony enlargement.
- No warmth on palpation.
- Erythrocyte sedimentation rate <40mm/hr.
- Rheumatoid factor <1:40.
- Osteophytes.
- Synovial fluid signs.

The NICE guidelines recommend only three clinical criteria together: age >45 years, pain related to activity, and stiffness of less than 30 minutes.

Management

Patient-centred care with an holistic approach is recommended by the NICE guidelines. Activity, continuing exercise and patient education are key to the management. Weight loss is recommended if the patient is obese.

Physical therapy

Regular muscle strengthening exercises are advised with general aerobic fitness. A physiotherapist can put together an individual structured plan for the patient.

Complementary therapies

Complementary therapies include heat and cold used locally as adjuncts. Also, many pain clinics use acupuncture and TENS machines successfully as part of the multimodal treatment.

Pharmacotherapy

Paracetamol and topical NSAIDs are recommended as first line by the NICE guidelines. A risk vs. benefit analysis is vital if any clinician is considering opioids especially in older people; if decided, these patients need a regular review for assessing the efficacy and outcomes. Topical capsaicin has a use as adjunctive therapy. An NSAID or a COX-2 selective inhibitor can be considered if other treatments do not help, but this should only be at the lowest effective dose for the shortest possible period. A gastric protective proton-pump inhibitor should always be prescribed alongside.

Injection therapy

Many pain clinics offer local injection treatments. Intra-articular injections also have a role if done appropriately.

Pain management programmes (PMPs)

PMPs can help in improving a patient's quality of life. Coping and pacing strategies are vital as in any chronic pain condition.

Surgery

A referral to a specialist surgeon is recommended if there is a prolonged and established functional limitation and severe pain.

Osteoporosis

Osteoporosis is a systemic disorder due to decreased bone mass, leading to bone fragility and an increased risks of fractures. It is more common in females. Osteoporosis affects more than 3 million people in the UK. More than 500,000 people in the UK receive hospital treatment for fragility fractures every year due to osteoporosis. Vertebral fractures are significant and cause long-term spinal pain.

Aetiopathology

Bone mass loss happens faster in some people causing osteopenia or osteoporosis; there is an imbalance between bone resorption and bone formation. Women lose bone rapidly after the start of menopause. High-dose steroid intake, family history, long-term hormonal medication intake (anti-oestrogen), obesity, lack of exercise, heavy drinking and smoking are associated risk factors.

Clinical features

Pain occurs only after a fracture. Some older patients may show bony changes in the spine even before the fracture.

Diagnosis

A bone density scan (dual-energy X-ray absorptiometry [DEXA] scan) calculates a T-score with standard deviation (SD). A SD between -1 and -2.5 is defined as osteopenia, and below -2.5 is classed as osteoporosis.

Management

Regular exercise, healthy eating and vitamin D can help in preventing osteoporosis.

Once diagnosed, the assessment of fragility fractures is vital. Online scoring systems such as FRAX® or QFracture® can be used. NICE recommends that adults who have a fragility fracture or use steroids or have a history of falls have an assessment of their fracture risk.

If symptomatic, non-pharmacological, complementary, pharmacological and injection treatments can be used as described in the previous section (see above: Osteoarthritis).

Medicines used to strengthen bones include:

- Bisphosphonates — slows the rate of breakdown of bone and maintains bone density (e.g. alendronate, zoledronate, risedronate).
- Calcium and vitamin D supplements.
- Other treatments — selective oestrogen receptor modulators, parathyroid hormone, hormone replacement therapy (in menopause), monoclonal antibody (denosumab).

An osteoporotic vertebral compression might need a percutaneous procedure such as a vertebroplasty or balloon kyphoplasty before considering surgical procedures.

Key Points

- Osteoarthritis is the most common joint disorder, due to multiple causes including loss of cartilage.
- Keeping active is the key to the management of osteoarthritis.
- NICE guidelines (CG177) for osteoarthritis recommend only three clinical criteria: age >45 years, pain related to activity, stiffness less than 30 minutes.
- Osteoporosis is due to decreased bone mass. A DEXA scan score below -2.5 is used in diagnosis.
- Fragility fractures are assessed using scoring systems such as FRAX® or Q-Fracture®.
- Bisphosphonates, calcium and vitamin D have a role to play in osteoporosis.

References

1.	Osteoarthritis-related pain. Global year against musculoskeletal pain 2009-2010. The International Association for the Study of Pain, 2017.

2.	Osteoarthritis: care and management. NICE clinical guideline, CG177. London: National Institute for Health and Care Excellence, 2014. https://www.nice.org.uk/guidance/cg177. Accessed on 6th July 2020.

3.	www.nhs.uk/conditions/osteoarthritis.

4.	Osteoporosis. Global year against musculoskeletal pain, 2009-2010. The International Association for the Study of Pain, 2017.

5.	www.nhs.uk/conditions/osteoporosis.

6.	Osteoporosis. NICE guidance, QS 149. London: National Institute for Health and Care Excellence, 2017. https://www.nice.org.uk/guidance/qs149. Accessed on 27th July 2020.

Chapter 8

Neuropathic pain

Shyam Balasubramanian

The definition of neuropathic pain is pain due to lesions or diseases involving the somatosensory nervous system.

Classification (■ Figure 8.1)

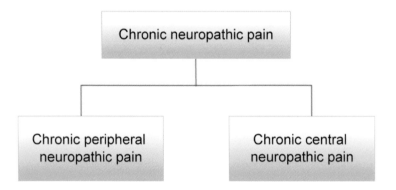

Figure 8.1. The classification of neuropathic pain.

Examples of chronic peripheral neuropathic pain are:

- Trigeminal neuralgia.
- Neuropathic pain following peripheral nerve injury (e.g. following surgery, trauma).
- Painful polyneuropathy (e.g. diabetes, alcoholism, B12 deficiency, infectious diseases, autoimmune diseases, chemotherapy-induced, idiopathic).
- Post-herpetic neuralgia.
- Painful (spinal) radiculopathy.

Examples of chronic central neuropathic pain are:

- Neuropathic pain following brain injury.
- Neuropathic pain following spinal cord injury.
- Chronic central post-stroke pain.
- Neuropathic pain associated with multiple sclerosis.

Mechanism

Changes can happen in the ascending pain pathway or in the descending inhibitory system. Some of the salient changes are described below.

Ascending pain pathway

Peripheral:

- Peripheral sensitization — inflammatory mediators such as substance P and calcitonin gene-related peptide (CGRP) are released, which in turn increase vascular permeability to byproducts of injury such as prostaglandins, growth factors, bradykinins and cytokines. These lower firing thresholds and cause ectopic discharges resulting in spontaneous pain.
- Ion channels — increased expression of sodium channels in the injured axon and dorsal root ganglia; increased expression of α2-delta-1 (α2-δ1) calcium channels in the dorsal root ganglia.

- Phenotypic switch — A-delta and C fibres transmit pain. Due to a phenotypic switch, other fibres can also release neurotransmitters such as substance P and CGRP.
- Sympathetically mediated pain — interaction between autonomic and somatosensory nerve fibres.

Spinal:

'Neuroplastic changes' take place along nociceptive pathways in the spinal and supraspinal regions:

- Activation of excitatory NMDA glutamate receptors.
- Glial cell activation — structural and functional changes in the glial cells following injury.
- Activation of spinal astrocytes.

Supraspinal:

- Changes in the regional concentration of neurotransmitters and metabolism happens in specific areas of the brain (e.g. thalamus, cingulate cortex).
- Patients with chronic pain may have reduced grey matter.

Descending inhibitory system

Spinal:

Ineffective descending inhibition due to:

- Dysfunctional GABA production and release.
- Decreased expression of μ-opioid receptors and a reduced response to opioids.
- Activation of excitatory NMDA glutaminergic receptors.

Supraspinal:

- The inhibitory neurotransmitters in the pathway are norepinephrine, serotonin, dopamine and opioids. Following nerve injury, there is a reduction in the effectiveness of the inhibitory pathway.

Assessment

History

- Site — dermatomal pattern, pain described in a specific nerve territory, glove and stocking distribution in metabolic neuropathies.
- Onset — insidious onset (metabolic neuropathy), post-surgical/post-traumatic.
- Character — pins and needles, burning, electric shock, shooting.
- Radiation — along the course of the nerve?
- Associated symptoms — depends on other underlying causes, e.g. multiple sclerosis.
- Time/duration — continuous/intermittent and recurrent?
- Exacerbating/relieving factors — e.g. hypersensitivity to touch, weather, specific movements.
- Severity — in mixed pain conditions, commonly, the neuropathic pain component is described as the most severe.

Examination

- Inspection — skin discolouration (sympathetically mediated pain), rashes (shingles), muscle wasting.
- Palpation:
  - positive sensory symptoms — allodynia (painful response to non-painful stimuli such as touch, pressure);
  - hyperalgesia (an exaggerated response to painful stimuli);
  - negative sensory symptoms — a decreased or loss of sensation.

Investigations

The choice of investigation is directed by the history and examination findings:

- Neurophysiology tests — to assess activity of the somatosensory nervous system (e.g. lateral femoral cutaneous nerve of the thigh for meralgia paraesthetica).
- Imaging studies — ultrasound or MRI scans to reveal anatomical changes that can lead to nerve dysfunction (e.g. spinal disc prolapse with compression on the nerve roots).
- Blood tests — for metabolic neuropathies, autoimmune disorders, nutritional deficiencies, endocrine abnormalities.
- Quantitative sensory testing (QST) — mainly a research tool and not commonly used in clinical practice.

Management

The management of neuropathic pain is multimodal and multidisciplinary with a biopsychosocial approach. The objectives are symptom relief and functional restoration. Treatment modalities include:

- Physical therapy.
- Pharmacotherapy.
- Injection therapy.
- Neuromodulation.
- Psychological interventions.
- Surgery.

Therapeutic management is challenging. Wherever possible, treat the cause (e.g. relieving the pressure on the nerve in compressive neuropathies; address the systemic factors in metabolic neuropathies).

Physical therapy

Range of movement, stretching and strengthening exercises and desensitization techniques can help patients with neuropathic pain.

Pharmacotherapy

- Antidepressants — amitriptyline, nortriptyline, duloxetine.
- Anticonvulsants — gabapentin, pregabalin, carbamazepine (trigeminal neuralgia).
- Transdermal patches — lidocaine, capsaicin.
- Opioids — tramadol, buprenorphine, etc. Some patients may respond to a stable, non-incremental dose of stronger opioids.

Injection therapy

- Axial (epidural), paraxial (paravertebral) and peripheral nerve blocks are used for diagnostic and therapeutic purposes.
- Intravenous lidocaine and magnesium infusions have a role in neuropathic pain.

Neuromodulation

When conventional interventions fail, neuromodulation techniques such as spinal cord or peripheral nerve stimulators can be used.

Psychological interventions

Cognitive behavioural therapy (CBT), acceptance and commitment therapy (ACT), mindfulness-based approaches, and pain management programmes (PMPs) can be helpful.

Surgery

Surgery is relevant for when there is structural irritation to the nerve, e.g. lumbar decompression surgery for radicular pain, carpal tunnel release.

Mechanism-based treatments are outlined in ■ Table 8.1.

Table 8.1. Mechanism-based treatments for neuropathic pain.

Peripheral — Lidocaine patch, capsaicin patch, menthol gel, peripheral nerve blocks, botulinum injections, peripheral nerve stimulation electrodes.

Spinal — Opioids, anticonvulsants, antidepressants, NMDA receptor antagonists, spinal injections (epidural, erector spinae plane block, etc.), spinal cord stimulation.

Supraspinal — Opioids, anticonvulsants, antidepressants, psychological interventions (CBT, etc.), deep brain stimulation.

Key Points

- Neuropathic pain is due to diseases or lesions involving the somatosensory nervous system.
- It can be central or peripheral.
- Assessment includes a history, an examination and investigations.
- Management is multimodal, directed at peripheral, spinal or supraspinal mechanisms.
- The goal is symptom relief and functional rehabilitation.

References

1. Scholz J, Finnerup NB, Attal N, *et al*. The IASP classification of chronic pain for ICD-11: Chronic neuropathic pain. *Pain* 2019; 160(1): 53-9.

2. Cohen SP, Mao J. Neuropathic pain: mechanisms and their clinical implications. *BMJ* 2014; 348: f7656.

3. Neuropathic pain in adults: pharmacological management in non-specialist settings. NICE clinical guideline, CG173. London: National Institute for Health and Care Excellence, 2013. https://www.nice.org.uk/guidance/cg173. Accessed on 6th July 2020.

Chapter 9

Complex regional pain syndrome

Thanthullu Vasu

Complex regional pain syndrome (CRPS) is a debilitating, painful condition with severe, continuous pain in the affected extremity, accompanied by sensory, vasomotor, sudomotor and motor/trophic changes. Pain is disproportionate to the initial injury. CRPS is more common in females, with a peak at the age of 40 years; it is more common in the upper extremities. The incidence is 20 to 26 per 100,000 people.

CRPS can be classified as Type I (without nerve injury) and Type II (with associated nerve injury).

Aetiopathology

There is a combination of peripheral and central nervous system involvement, but the exact pathophysiology is not clearly understood.

Peripheral pathophysiological mechanisms include: an abnormality in primary afferents (spontaneous discharge, sensitization, ectopic sensitivity); sodium channel spontaneous discharge; C nociceptor norepinephrine responsiveness; neurogenic inflammatory reaction (increased CGRP and substance P); small fibre neuropathy and tissue hypoxia.

Central mechanisms include: spinal cord hyperexcitability; dynamic hyperexcitability in central neurons; changes in somatosensory mapping in the brain; NMDA-mediated hyperexcitability in the dorsal horn; somatosensory sensitization; central sympathetic vasoconstrictor inhibition.

Theories of sympathetic system involvement have been put forward to explain the symptoms. The autoimmune theory proposes an auto-antibody mediated response. Inflammatory mediators including interleukins are proposed but the theories are still unclear. Deep tissue microvascular ischaemia and reperfusion injury is proposed as another hypothesis. Genetic factors may be involved in the predisposition of CRPS (specific HLA antigen-related).

Clinical features

- Sensory signs and symptoms — burning pain, neuropathic features.
- Autonomic abnormalities — swelling, oedema, vasomotor changes, skin temperature changes, changes in sweating.
- Trophic changes in later stages — nail and hair growth, skin changes, bone changes including osteoporosis.
- Motor changes — weakness, neurological changes, neglect-like symptoms in the affected extremity.

Diagnosis

The Budapest criteria are used in the diagnosis of CRPS:

- Pain should be continuous and disproportionate to the initial event.
- At least one sign in two or more categories.
- At least one symptom in three or more categories.
- No other diagnosis exists to explain the symptoms of pain.

The categories are:

- Sensory — allodynia, hyperalgesia, hyperaesthesia.
- Vasomotor — temperature (more than 1°C) or skin colour asymmetry in limbs.
- Sudomotor — sweating changes, oedema.
- Motor/trophic — decreased range of motion, motor dysfunction, hair/nail/skin trophic changes.

Two signs and three symptoms in different categories are needed for a diagnosis, as explained above.

Management

Early recognition and treatment are essential. Physiotherapy (gradual exercises) and rehabilitation are the key to recovery. Early mobilisation with adequate pain relief is vital in long-term recovery. Desensitization and education play a big role in patient understanding and engagement with the treatment.

Physical therapy

Graded exercises are recommended.

Complementary therapies

TENS machines and acupuncture are used in many pain clinics.

Pharmacotherapy

Neuropathics are used commonly if appropriate which require a review for their efficacy and side effects (see Chapter 8 on Neuropathic pain and the various chapters on pharmacology).

Occupational therapy

Laterality recognition, graded motor imagery, etc., help with central mechanisms; mirror box therapy has been used successfully.

Injection therapy

Sympathetic blocks have been tried. Intravenous regional blocks can be used as part of multimodal treatment. Various regional blocks have been used to engage patients in gradual rehabilitation.

Neuromodulation

Spinal cord stimulation can be considered if other treatments do not help.

Psychological interventions

Multidisciplinary team management, and coping and pacing skills are included as needed in all patients. Pain management programmes have a role in recovery if these treatments do not help.

Other treatments

Other treatments include bisphosphonates (alendronate, IV palmidronate), botulinium toxin injections, calcium modulating drugs, free radical scavengers, vitamin C and corticosteroids.

Key Points

- CRPS — disproportionate pain with sensory, vasomotor, sudomotor and motor/trophic changes.
- Budapest criteria: at least two signs and three symptoms in different categories.
- Early recognition, physiotherapy and rehabilitation are vital.
- Desensitization is the key to recovery.

References

1.   Bharwani KD, Dirckx M, Huygen FJPM. Complex regional pain syndrome: diagnosis and treatment. *BJA Educ* 2017; 17(8): 262-8.

2.   CRPS in adults. UK guidelines for diagnosis, referral and management in primary and secondary care. Royal College of Physicians, 2018.

3.   Charlton JE. *Core curriculum for professional education in pain.* IASP Press, 2005.

Chapter 10

Fibromyalgia

Thanthullu Vasu

Functional pain syndromes do not have a physiological or organic cause for the pain despite extensive investigations. They include a spectrum of conditions that can sometimes coexist: fibromyalgia, pelvic pain, irritable bowel and bladder, chronic fatigue, temporomandibular joint problems, etc.

Fibromyalgia is characterised by chronic, diffuse musculoskeletal pain and tenderness with associated symptoms including sleep disturbances, fatigue and affective dysfunction. It affects 2-10% of the population and is seen more in females (seven times more common than males).

Aetiopathology

It is not clear but various theories are proposed:

- Neurosensory — central pain amplification, central sensitization, abnormalities in the descending inhibitory pathway.
- Neurotransmitter — reduced serotonin in pain pathways centrally, elevated substance P and nerve growth factor in CSF, NMDA-related wind-up.
- Neuroendocrine — dysfunction of hypothalamic-pituitary-adrenal axis, abnormal cortisol response and growth hormone.
- Genetic — familial tendency, genetic polymorphisim in serotoninergic, dopaminergic and catecholaminergic systems.
- Environmental stressors can act as triggering factors, e.g. trauma, infection.

Diagnosis and clinical features

The recent American College of Rheumatology (ACR) (2010) guidelines does not rely on the previously used less sensitive method of assessing tender points. It uses the Widespread Pain Index (WPI) and Symptom Severity (SS) scale and assigns a score.

Three conditions are required:

- WPI ≥7 and SS ≥5 (or WPI 3-6 and SS ≥9).
- Symptoms of more than 3 months.
- No other disorder that could explain the pain.

WPI — 19 areas in the body where the pain occurred in the last week; score of 0-19.

SS — fatigue, waking unrefreshed, cognitive symptoms, extent of somatic symptoms (each scored 0-3), giving a total of 0-12.

Investigations

Blood tests are needed to rule out other causes; sinister red flags have to be ruled out. Fibromyalgia is a clinical diagnosis based on the ACR criteria (as mentioned above) after ruling out causes.

Management

Fibromyalgia can significantly affect the quality of life of a patient and requires a multimodal biopsychosocial model of pain management. Education is vital for the patient and family to make sure that they understand the pathophysiology and the need to look at a biopsychosocial model of pain management. The diagnosis and explanation forms a key to the comprehensive management plan. The aim should be to improve quality of life and function.

Many of these patients have already visited multiple specialist clinics without a proper diagnosis; thus, it is important to strike a good rapport, explain everything in detail and gain the confidence of the patient to avoid the 'revolving door' phenomenon of repeated clinical consults and investigations.

Physical therapy

Aerobic and strengthening exercises — there is level I evidence to support their use.

Complementary therapies

Complementary therapies include:

- Acupuncture — there is level I evidence to support this therapy.
- Hydrotherapy has been used with good evidence.
- A TENS machine can achieve some success along with patient education.
- Yoga and tai-chi can be used to improve function.

Pharmacotherapy

- Neuropathics (see the relevant chapters on neuropathic medications).
- Weak opioids such as tramadol can be used but a risk assessment and review are vital.
- Cyclobenzaprine is suggested but is not used in the UK.

Invasive treatments

An intravenous lignocaine infusion has a limited effect but is used to improve the quality of life in a multimodal approach in many pain services.

Psychological interventions

- Cognitive behavioural therapies (CBTs) — there is level I evidence to support CBT.
- Mindfulness-based therapy and acceptance-commitment therapy (ACT) have been successfully used in many pain services.

Pain management programmes

The patient needs to be referred to a PMP if their quality of life is poor.

Key Points

- Functional pain syndromes present as a spectrum of diseases with no clear diagnosis.
- The ACR 2010 guidelines for the diagnosis of fibromyalgia are:
  - WPI ≥7 and SS ≥5 (or WPI 3-6 and SS ≥9);
  - symptoms more than 3 months;
  - no other disorder that could explain the pain.
- Multimodal comprehensive management is based upon biopsychosocial principles.
- It is important to educate and gain the confidence of the patient so that he/she can engage with the treatment pathway.

References

1. Fibromyalgia. IASP. Global year against musculoskeletal pain 2009-2010. The International Association for the Study of Pain, 2017.

2. Wolfe F, Clauw DJ, Fitzcharles M-A, *et al.* The American College of Rheumatology preliminary diagnostic criteria for fibromyalgia and measurement of symptom severity. *Arthritis Care Res* 2010; 62(5): 600-10.

3. Macfarlane G, Kronish C, Dean LE, *et al.* EULAR revised recommendations for the management of fibromyalgia. *Ann Rheum Dis* 2017; 76(2): 318-28.

Chapter 11

Rheumatological considerations

Thanthullu Vasu

Rheumatoid arthritis

Rheumatoid arthritis is a chronic systemic inflammatory autoimmune disease that affects the synovium of the joints. It affects 0.5% of the population and is more common in women; the peak age is 65-74 years. The risk is increased with a family history of the disease and in smokers.

Clinical features

Symmetrical polyarticular inflammation of the joints presents as pain, swelling and stiffness. It is common in the joints of hands, wrists and feet. Joint destruction leads to functional limitations.

Extra-articular features include: nodules, osteoporosis, vasculitis, lung fibrosis, neuropathy.

Other features include: morning stiffness, fatigue, sweating.

Diagnosis

The American College of Rheumatology/European League Against Rheumatism (2010) classification outlines scores of more than or equal to 6 from:

- Joint involvement (0-5).

- Serology (rheumatoid factor, anti-citrullinated antibodies) (0-3).
- Acute phase reactants (CRP, ESR) (0-1).
- Duration of symptoms — 6 weeks (0-1).

Management

- Multimodal pain management with a focus on physiotherapy and occupational therapy is needed.
- Non-steroidal anti-inflammatory drugs are standard treatment for rheumatoid arthritis. These help symptoms but do not alter the progression of the disease.
- Disease-modifying antirheumatic drugs (DMARDs) reduce the damage and act by cytokine inhibition, reducing damage done to the joints:
  - older drugs such as sulfasalazine produce a slow response and are toxic;
  - methotrexate improves inflammation but is needed long term;
  - newer DMARDs: TNF-α antagonists — monoclonal antibodies — inhibit structural damage to joints, e.g. infliximab, etanercept, golimumab.
- Corticosteroids — reduce joint damage, but there is a need to monitor for side effects (cardiovascular, osteoporosis).
- Other drugs — anakinra (human recombinant IL-1 antagonist), rituximab (depletes B cells), tocilizumab (human monoclonal IL-6 antagonist).

Chronic fatigue syndrome

Chronic fatigue syndrome is a severe disabling fatigue, associated with pain, sleep disturbance, impaired concentration, etc. The prevalence ranges from 0.2 to 0.4% and is more common in females, age 20-40 years. This was termed by some in the past as myalgic encephalomyelitis (ME).

Aetiopathology

A number of mechansims have been proposed including: genetic, immunologic, infections, endocrine (HPA axis) and psychosocial factors.

Clinical features

Fatigue, malaise, sleep disturbances, headaches, difficulty in concentration.

Management

Patient-centred care should take into account the needs of the individual. Gradual paced exercises and cognitive behavioural therapy have shown good evidence of being effective. The aim is to improve quality of life.

Connective tissue diseases

A variety of diseases can affect connective tissues in the body, ranging from:

- Congential — Marfan syndrome, Ehlers-Danlos syndrome, osteogenesis imperfecta.
- Autoimmune — systemic lupus erythematosus, rheumatoid arthritis, scleroderma, mixed connective tissue disease.

Key Points

- Rheumatoid arthritis — a chronic systemic inflammatory autoimmune disease that affects the synovium of the joints.
- NSAIDs, DMARDs, newer DMARDs and steroids have a role to play in rheumatoid arthritis.

References

1.   Emery P. Treatment of rheumatoid arthritis. *BMJ* 2006; 332: 152-5.

2.   Klarenbeek NB, Kerstens PJSM, Huizinga TWJ, *et al.* Recent advances in the management of rheumatoid arthritis. *BMJ* 2010; 341: c6942.

3.   Reid S, Chalder T, Cleare A, *et al.* Chronic fatigue syndrome. *BMJ* 2000; 320: 292.

4.   Chronic fatigue syndrome/myalgic encephalomyelitis (or encephalopathy): diagnosis and management. NICE clinical guideline, CG53. London: National Institute for Health and Care Excellence, 2007. https://www.nice.org.uk/guidance/cg53. Accessed on 6th July 2020.

Chapter 12

Painful diabetic neuropathy

Pradeep Mukund Ingle

Painful diabetic neuropathy (PDN) is a disabling condition due to abnormalities in the somatosensory nervous system causing pain, usually in the periphery of the extremities secondary to diabetes mellitus.

Diabetes is the most common cause of peripheral neuropathy in the UK. Interestingly, peripheral neuropathy is amongst the most common complication of diabetes and it causes pain in more than half of those with this neuropathy.

Risk factors

The EURODIAB IDDM Complications Study carried out in 16 European countries noted that the prevalence of diabetic peripheral neuropathy was 28% in Europe with no significant differences geographically. This correlated with some factors which increased the risk:

- Duration of diabetes.
- Advancing age.
- Quality of metabolic control — poor diabetic control/high HbA1c levels.
- Cigarette smoking.
- High BMI.
- Presence of diabetic retinopathy.
- Presence of cardiovascular disease, e.g. hypertension.
- High-density lipoprotein cholesterol/hypertriglyceridaemia.

Classification

- Generalised symmetrical polyneuropathies — chronic sensorimotor peripheral polyneuropathy. The commonest type is purely sensory or a mixed type; acute sensory painful polyneuropathy; autonomic neuropathy.
- Focal polyneuropathies.

Aetiopathology

The exact cause is complex and not completely understood but the initiation of this process is linked with a hyperglycemic state causing accumulation of glycosylated end products with neuronal injury. This process can be explained as follows:

- Generation of glycosylated end products around the peripheral nerves and capillaries reduces nerve conduction velocity. Arteriopathy-related ischaemic damage also affects nerve conduction.
- Increased oxidative stress leading to oxidative free radical formation.
- Calcium and sodium channel dysfunction causing neuronal hyperexcitability.
- Lower levels of insulin-like growth factors and neuronal growth factors lead to impaired regeneration of the neurons.
- Increased neuronal excitability at the synapse can lead to NMDA receptor-mediated central sensitization.
- By recruitment of multiple subthreshold inputs, central sensitization augments noxious and non-noxious stimuli causing neuropathic pain.

Clinical manifestations

Sensory neuropathy affects touch, pain and temperature conducting fibres along with loss of kinaesthetic, proprioceptive and vibration sensations. It can also lead to tingling and numbness in the affected area with features of neuropathic pain in the distribution of the nerves. This makes it prone to injury in that region leading to complications such as ulcers typically seen in areas such as the feet. Rarely, severe sensory neuropathy can lead to complications such as Charcot joints.

Motor neuropathy can lead to muscle wasting and weakness, muscle twitching and cramps along with an inability to perform motor tasks such as handling of small objects, fastening of buttons and going up staircases. Motor neuropathy in the lower limbs or feet can result in a loss of coordination with altered gait. This can make patients more prone to foot injuries.

Autonomic neuropathy affects the cardiovascular system, genitourinary system and gastrointestinal system. This can result in various clinical manifestations such as diabetic gastroparesis, loss of bladder control, cardiac autonomic neuropathy (leading to loss of beat to beat variability with resting tachycardia which increases the risk of arrhythmias and sudden death), poor temperature regulation due to impaired sweating and erectile dysfunction. Autonomic neuropathy can lead to trophic changes (such as dry feet, callous formations, abnormal nail/hair growth), vasomotor changes (colour changes in the feet including pale, red or blue and temperature changes) and sudomotor changes (altered sweating and swelling) over the skin.

Clinical features can include numbness and pain in the feet extending up to the leg and sometimes the hands (glove and stalking type of distribution which is typical). Pain can worsen at night with disturbed sleep and mood, and can affect quality of life.

Signs can include reduced sensations to touch, pain (pin prick), temperature, vibrations and proprioception; and reduced reflexes such as ankle and knee jerk reflexes.

Differential diagnoses

Nutritional/vitamin deficiencies, structural neural compressions/lesions, degenerative conditions, endocrine disorders, and vascular, toxic, immune-mediated and infective causes need to be ruled out as appropriate. They may coexist with diabetic polyneuropathy as well.

Investigations

Investigations are usually undertaken to identify the treatable causes and not for diagnosing PDN. They include electrodiagnostic tests (EMG and NCS), nerve biopsy and quantitative sensory testing (in research settings only).

Management

The management of painful diabetic neuropathy is with multidisciplinary management using a biopsychosocial approach comprising non-pharmacological, pharmacological and interventional strategies. Educating patients on glycaemic control and its need is vital which can be done with appropriate communication skills in the pain clinic.

Prevention

- Optimisation of diabetes control and regular checks for peripheral neuropathy.
- Optimisation of comorbidities and risk factors.
- Early involvement of the diabetic foot care team and referral to a pain clinic as per the NICE guidelines.

Physical therapy

Physiotherapy for feet and appropriate foot care management.

Complementary therapies

It is important to ensure good sleep hygiene. Alternative therapies and complementary medications may be tried including acupuncture and TENS.

Pharmacotherapy

Usually neuropathic pain does not respond to simple analgesics such as paracetamol and NSAIDs. In accordance with the NICE guidelines for the management of neuropathic pain, this involves a combination of oral and topical medications. (See Chapter 8 on Neuropathic pain and the relevant chapters on pharmacology.)

Lignocaine 5% plasters can be considered for localised pain. A capsaicin patch 8% is licensed for peripheral neuropathic pain. A single application for 30 minutes can yield benefit for more than 3 months.

Injection therapy

Regional blocks provide a short-term benefit usually, but they can be part of a multimodal comprehensive plan.

Neuromodulation

Interventional approaches (limited evidence) include:

- Spinal cord stimulation.
- Peripheral nerve stimulation and dorsal root ganglion stimulation.

Psychological interventions

Optimizing treatment of other coexisting conditions such as anxiety, depression, etc., is important, along with psychology-based interventions such as CBT and ACT as needed.

Key Points

- Painful diabetic neuropathy (PDN) is a very common cause of pain in diabetic patients and is often managed suboptimally.
- Management of its risk factors is vital in minimising the progression of neuropathic pain.
- PDN can be sensory, motor, mixed or autonomic in its presentation.
- The optimal management of PDN involves a holistic multidisciplinary approach.

References

1. Rajan RS, de Gray L, George E. Painful diabetic neuropathy. *Contin Educ Anaesth Crit Care Pain* 2014; 14(5): 230-5.
2. Arora N, Niraj G. Management of painful peripheral diabetic neuropathy. *BJMP* 2013; 6(1): a606.
3. https://www.diabetes.org.uk/guide-to-diabetes/complications/nerves_neuropathy.
4. Azhary H, Farooq MU, Bhanushali M, *et al*. Peripheral neuropathy: differential diagnosis and management. *Am Fam Physician* 2010; 81(7): 887-92.
5. Colloca L, Ludman T, Bouhassira D, *et al*. Neuropathic pain. *Nat Rev Dis Primers* 2017; 3: 17002.

Chapter 13

Post-herpetic neuralgia

Pradeep Mukund Ingle

Pain lasting for more than 3 months following a *Herpes zoster* infection in one or more sensory dermatomal distributions along with skin changes is called post-herpetic neuralgia (PHN).

Aetiopathology

Varicella zoster virus infection (chicken pox) is common in childhood; the virus persists in a clinically latent form in spinal and cranial sensory nerves, sensory dorsal root ganglia and at the dorsal horn level. The reactivation of this latent form results in shingles, which presents as a rash over the affected dermatomes along with associated pain. After a few days or sometimes weeks, the painful area develops acute vesicular eruption in the affected dermatomes. Necrosis and inflammation of the skin in affected dermatomes occur during this phase of viral replication. The proposed mechanism of PHN includes various changes in the neurons that are responsible for the long-term pain:

- At the spinal cord level, it is associated with primary afferent neuronal degeneration along with atrophy of the dorsal horn and dorsal root ganglion scarring which causes denervation of the dermatomal region over the skin.
- Demyelinated Aβ fibres can spontaneously discharge (abnormally) leading to spontaneous pain paroxysms.
- A combination of neural injury and inflammation can lead to peripheral sensitization increasing the afferent input to the spinal cord.

- Also, sprouting of Aβ fibres centrally secondary to the reduction of C fibre inputs can lead to central sensitization.
- Allodynia and hyperalgesia result from regenerating Aβ fibres that connect with central receptors which would have otherwise normally received input from the C fibres.

Shingles and pain progression

Pain arising from the reactivation of *Herpes* (shingles) can be acute (<30 days of onset of rash), subacute (30-120 days) or can develop into chronic post-herpetic neuralgia (pain for at least 120 days after the rash begins). However, not all cases of shingles lead to PHN (only around 20% lead to PHN).

Shingles is uncommon at <15 years of age and is more common in those over 50 years of age, with its incidence rising with age significantly more in the elderly. It is more common in patients with reduced cell-mediated immunity which includes the elderly, patients with HIV infection, active cancer or those on chemotherapeutic drugs or radiotherapy, and patients on corticosteroid treatments, etc.

Risk factors for severe pain include a more severe rash and psychosocial factors such as poor coping skills and anxiety.

Clinical presentation

Shingles is usually preceded by a prodromal period with pain and abnormal skin sensations followed by a rash (usually vesicular) afterwards that resembles localised chicken pox in the dermatomal distribution. It usually involves one or two dermatomes and is unilateral.

Thoracic and abdominal dermatomes are affected more commonly although the ophthalmic division of the trigeminal nerve can be affected as well. It can also affect the genitals and other areas over the face. In immunocompromised people, the disease can be widespread with a severe and longlasting rash. Hospitalisation may be needed in systemically unwell patients with shingles.

In PHN, the pain in affected dermatomes stays for more than 3 months. PHN pain can be constant or intermittent; it can be spontaneous or evoked. It is usually neuropathic pain with features such as allodynia and hyperalgesia. This causes pain to start, with even a minimal stimulus such as from light touch or even by brushing of the patient's own clothes against the skin. As a result, any physical activity can potentially cause pain due to the dermatomal stimulus. Usually the pain is sharp and aching in nature with neuropathic features such as throbbing, burning, electric shock-like or lancinating.

Sleep interference is very common along with other associated features such as anxiety, depression, chronic fatigue, weight loss and a difficulty in focusing, which has a negative impact on QOL.

Affected sensations in the dermatome are unilateral. They include temperature, vibration, touch and pinprick sensations. Skin scarring and pigmentation along with itching and a sensory deficit are common features in the affected dermatomes.

Usually pain improves in >50% patients of PHN at 6 months and they will need minimal or no treatment. However, some cases progress to severe long-term pain and they can be very difficult to treat.

Differential diagnoses

Differential diagnoses include: *Herpes simplex* infection, contact dermatitis, other causes of dermatomal neuropathic pain including radiculopathies, traumatic lesions in peripheral nerves, trigeminal neuralgia and trigeminal neuropathic pain.

Investigations

This is a clinical diagnosis based on history and examination, and usually no investigations are needed. Rarely, to differentiate the subtypes of *Herpes* virus, some investigations such as viral cultures, immunofluorescent staining and specific antibody testing may be done. QST is helpful to quantify the sensory loss in terms of thresholds but is useful for research purposes mainly and is rarely done in clinical practice.

Management

Preventive approaches for PHN

- A vaccine to prevent primary varicella (against chicken pox) can be administered to children to reduce the incidence of chicken pox and in turn subsequent zoster infection.
- A second type of vaccine for shingles (zoster vaccine) can be offered to people over 70 years of age to boost their immunity against zoster. This is usually offered in the UK to the elderly population. It reduces the severity of shingles and progression to PHN in this age group.
- Oral antivirals (acyclovir, valaciclovir or famciclovir) should be considered during the acute phase of shingles within 72 hours of the rash in high-risk populations such as immunocompromised patients, shingles with non-truncal involvement and those with a moderate to severe rash and pain. Antivirals help in reducing the severity of infection and pain, along with hastening the healing process. They should also be considered within 72 hours of a rash in patients >50 years of age to reduce the progression to PHN, although the evidence for this practice is not strong.
- Short courses of corticosteroids during the acute phase of zoster infection are commonly used clinically, but are unlikely to prevent progression to PHN.
- Severe pain in the acute phase of shingles can be managed with the addition of anti-neuropathic medications to minimise it progressing to chronic pain (weak evidence).

Pain management for PHN

Multidisciplinary team management incorporating a biopsychosocial model involving pharmacological, non-pharmacological and interventional approaches must be used for managing PHN.

Severe pain in PHN with limitations in activities of daily living should involve specialist services such as pain management referral.

Regular follow-up as needed to assess the progress of the condition, to understand the effectiveness, adverse effects and tolerability of current medications must be done in PHN patients.

Physical therapy

Measures to reduce skin irritation such as loose clothing, and covering the skin area with cling film or cold/ice packs (if no allodynia) can be utilised with varying benefits.

A TENS machine can be tried at the dermatomal level also.

Pharmacotherapy

Multimodal analgesic management is likely to be more effective:

- Mild to moderate pain — by simple analgesics such as paracetamol combined with codeine.
- Poorly controlled neuropathic pain needs management with anti-neuropathic drugs in accordance with NICE guidance involving amitriptyline, nortriptyline, gabapentinoids or duloxetine. Switching between anti-neuropathic drugs based on their effectiveness and tolerability must be done as per NICE guidelines.
- Consider topical measures such as capsaicin cream (0.075% cream), a capsaicin patch 8%, and lidocaine 5% plasters in patients who are not able to tolerate anti-neuropathic medications (e.g. frail elderly patients at risk of CNS side effects which can be significant) or in severe pain as an adjunct to the anti-neuropathic medications. They can be used as a sole agent in mild to moderate pain if tolerated and found to be effective.
- Tramadol can be used as an acute short-term rescue therapy only. Other opioids can be helpful in pain management initially but are not recommended for long-term management of chronic non-malignant pain in view of their potential for long-term side effects.

Injection therapy

There is limited evidence for injection therapies such as local infiltrations, peripheral nerve blocks, nerve root blocks, dorsal root ganglion injections, sympathetic blocks, and epidural and intrathecal injections with local anaesthetics and corticosteroids. Most of these procedures result in short-term pain relief which some patients may find useful.

Neuromodulation

Although spinal cord stimulation has a role in chronic neuropathic pain, its use specifically for PHN is backed by a limited number of studies showing efficacy. This needs to be explored further to assess its actual long-term benefits in PHN patients.

Psychological interventions

Any associated underlying psychological conditions such as depression need optimising. Psychology services can be utilised for CBT or ACT.

Key Points

- Activation of the varicella zoster virus (latent chicken pox) infection results in *Herpes zoster* infection or shingles.
- PHN is pain lasting for more than 3 months following a *Herpes zoster* infection (shingles) in one or more sensory dermatomal distributions along with skin changes.
- Although pain in most cases of PHN settles on its own at 6 months, some may progress to severe disabling chronic pain which responds poorly to medical management and this affects QOL significantly.
- Multidisciplinary team management for severe PHN using a combination of pharmacological, non-pharmacological and interventional approaches is the key to optimise pain management.

References

1.   Gupta R, Smith PF. Post-herpetic neuralgia. *Contin Educ Anaesth Critical Care Pain* 2012; 12(4): 181-5.

2.   https://cks.nice.org.uk/post-herpetic-neuralgia.

3.   Han Y, Zhang J, Chen N. Corticosteroids for preventing postherpetic neuralgia. *Cochrane Database Syst Rev* 2013. Available at: https://doi.org/10.1002/14651858.CD005582.pub4.

4.   https://cks.nice.org.uk/shingles.

5.   Nalamachu S, Morley-Forster P. Diagnosing and managing postherpetic neuralgia. *Drugs Aging* 2012; 29(11): 863-9.

Chapter 14

Chronic post-surgical pain (CPSP)

Mahesh Kodivalasa

The International Association for the Study of Pain (IASP) classifies chronic post-surgical pain as a secondary chronic pain condition in the WHO International Classification of Diseases (ICD-11).

Chronic post-surgical pain (CPSP) is defined as chronic pain that develops or increases in intensity after a surgical procedure or a tissue injury and persists beyond the healing process, i.e. at least 3 months after the surgery or tissue trauma. The new definition brings some uniformity and clarity in reporting the incidence of chronic post-surgical pain after various surgical procedures.

The cumulative overall incidence varies from as low as 5% to as high as 85%. Thoracotomy, sternotomy, mastectomy, cholecystectomy, inguinal hernia repair, and limb amputation are a few of the surgical procedures known to have a high incidence (ranging above 50%).

Although various risk factors for the development of chronic post-surgical pain have been identified, not all the factors are modifiable. Non-modifiable risk factors include age, sex, genetic susceptibility, location of trauma/pathology. Females in younger age groups are more susceptible. Pre-operative modifiable risk factors include continuous or severe pre-operative pain, other chronic pain conditions and psychosocial factors. Intra-operative modifiable risk factors include the duration of surgery, extent of tissue damage, nerve damage and repeat surgery.

Nerve damage with shearing force is hypothesised as a more important cause than a clean-cut deliberate injury. It is important to note that not all chronic post-surgical pain conditions are neuropathic in nature and not all nerve injuries lead to neuropathic pain.

Postoperative risk factors include severe and prolonged postoperative pain. Peri-operative radiotherapy is also shown to be a risk factor.

The main proposed pathophysiological mechanisms for the development of chronic post-surgical pain include peripheral and central sensitization. Tissue/nerve injury releases inflammatory and immune mediators. These mediators lower the firing threshold and raise the firing potential of peripheral nociceptors in addition to recruiting dormant nociceptors. Continuous and repetitive ascending pain signals in the central pathways lead to neuroplastic changes responsible for the maintenance of a chronic pain state. NMDA receptors and microglial cells play a significant role.

Preventive strategies

- Identification of patients at risk.
- Multidisciplinary approach.
- Patient education and psychological preparation.
- Minimally invasive surgery where possible.
- Nerve-sparing surgery.
- Modified anaesthetic techniques incorporating regional anaesthesia and analgesia.
- Multimodal analgesic regimens.
- The peri-operative use of gabapentinoids, ketamine, clonidine and intravenous lidocaine has shown some evidence in preventing chronic post-surgical pain.

Management

- Multidisciplinary — a biopsychosocial approach.
- Pharmacological — multimodal analgesia with anti-neuropathic medications as the mainstay of therapy.
- Topical therapies may include capsaicin and local anaesthetic patches.

- Complementary therapies have very weak evidence for their use.
- Interventional management options include scar infiltration, peripheral nerve blocks, neuraxial blocks (epidural and paravertebral blocks), sympathectomies, fascial plane blocks (transversus abdominis plane, rectus, quadratus lumborum, serratus plane block), IV lidocaine, etc.
- Peripheral and neuraxial neuromodulation.

Key Points

- CPSP is pain that persists after a healing period, i.e. 3 months.
- Modifiable and non-modifiable risk factors have been identified.
- Peripheral and central sensitization is the proposed theory behind CPSP.
- Multimodal analgesia with regional blocks during the peri-operative period can reduce the incidence of CPSP.

References

1. Thapa P, Euasobhon P. Chronic postsurgical pain: current evidence for prevention and management. *Korean J Pain* 2018; 31(3): 155-73.

2. Richebé P, Capdevila X, Rivat C. Persistent postsurgical pain: pathophysiology and preventative pharmacologic considerations. *Anesthesiology* 2018; 129(3): 590-607.

3. Searle RD, Simpson KH. Chronic post-surgical pain. *Contin Educ Anaesth Critical Care Pain* 2010; 10(1): 12-4.

Chapter 15

Prevention of chronic post-surgical pain

Mahesh Kodivalasa

Evidence clearly exists to prove that the proper peri-operative management of acute pain can reduce the incidence and severity of chronic pain. It is prudent that the anaesthetist and surgical team use multimodal analgesia with regional blocks during the peri-operative period wherever possible.

Pre-emptive analgesia and preventive analgesia

Pre-emptive analgesia

- Pre-emptive analgesia is given prior to an injury or noxious stimulus.
- The focus of pre-emptive analgesia is on the timing of an intervention, i.e. before or after an incision.
- The concept is based on the principle that a nociceptive barrage from the site of injury induces secondary changes leading to central sensitization. Abolition of this initiating event prevents secondary changes and thereby reduces the incidence of ongoing chronic post-surgical pain.
- The clinical usefulness of pre-emptive analgesia is disappointing. The research evidence is weak and contradictory.
- One of the possible reasons is that the concept of prevention of central sensitization with a single timed intervention — thereby preventing or reducing ongoing pain — is too simple. A nociceptive barrage continues throughout surgery.
- In addition, the other problem associated with the study of the effect of pre-emptive analgesia is that research methodologies included varied study designs and outcome measures.

Preventive analgesia

- Preventive analgesia is a peri-operative intervention incorporating the administration of analgesia prior to, during, and after the noxious stimulus.
- In preventive analgesia the focus is on the effect of the intervention on the expected duration of analgesia and prevention of central sensitization. This is regardless of when the intervention takes place in relation to surgery (time insensitive).
- Preventive analgesia is a broader concept compared with pre-emptive analgesia.
- Preventive analgesia acknowledges the fact that multiple factors are involved in central sensitization after an acute noxious event such as surgery.
- There are mainly two phases to the noxious surgical stimulus: the primary phase is related to the surgery itself and the secondary phase involves chemicals and inflammatory mediators released from the damaged tissue. The secondary phase begins in the intra-operative period and extends into the postoperative period.
- Preventive analgesia is based on the principle that a nociceptive barrage leads to central sensitization which continues throughout the peri-operative period. A mechanism of minimising or blocking this continuous noxious sensory input prevents central sensitization.
- Multimodal preventive analgesic regimens have synergistic effects thus reducing postoperative pain and the overall requirements of analgesic medications. The regimens may include a combination of oral, systemic and regional techniques in the peri-operative period.
- A preventive analgesic regimen may consist of:
  - pre-operative paracetamol, NSAIDs and gabapentinoids;
  - intra-operative opioids, regional blocks or infusions and systemic infusions comprising lidocaine or magnesium or ketamine;
  - postoperative continuation of systemic and regional infusions along with other medications.
- If an agent/intervention is capable of reducing sensitization, then its effects would be expected to extend beyond its normal duration of action. This may or may not be related to the timing of administration.

- An analgesic is said to have a preventive effect if its administration leads to a reduction in pain or analgesic consumption that extends beyond its expected duration of action (usually set at 5.5 half-lives).
- Evidence shows that preventive analgesia can lead to better recovery, early discharge from hospital, improved function, better patient satisfaction and a reduced incidence of chronic post-surgical pain.

Key Points

- The focus of pre-emptive analgesia is on the timing of an intervention.
- Preventive analgesia is a broader concept compared with pre-emptive analgesia and is time-insensitive.
- The evidence for pre-emptive analgesia is weak and contradictory.
- The evidence shows better outcomes with preventive analgesia.

References

1.   Shah AC, Nair BG, Spiekerman CF, Bollag LA. Continuous intraoperative epidural infusions affect recovery room length of stay and analgesic requirements: a single-center observational study. *J Anesth* 2017; 31(4): 494-501.

2.   Rosero EB, Joshi GP. Preemptive, preventive, multimodal analgesia. *Plast Reconstruct Surg* 2014; 134(4S-2): 85S-93S.

3.   Lavand'homme P. From preemptive to preventive analgesia: time to reconsider the role of perioperative peripheral nerve blocks? *Reg Anesth Pain Med* 2011; 36(1): 4-6.

Chapter 16

Post-amputation pain

Shyam Balasubramanian

The term 'post-amputation pain' includes a myriad of presentations of variable aetiopathogenesis. The prevalence is high, and the management is challenging.

Presentation (■ Figure 16.1)

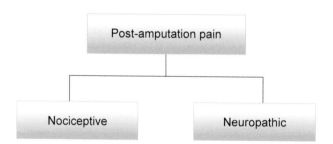

Figure 16.1. Presentations of post-amputation pain.

Nociceptive pain includes: myofascial pain (from muscles), a bony spur, an ill-fitting prosthesis, chronic infection (in the soft tissues, osteomyelitis), vascular causes (ischaemia), musculoskeletal pain in other areas secondary to biomechanical changes (in the back, opposite limb, etc).

Neuropathic pain includes: phantom pain (pain in the part of the limb that is missing), and stump neuropathic pain (pain in the residual limb).

These different pain conditions often coexist.

Aetiopathology

The aetiopathology has supraspinal, spinal and peripheral mechanisms (refer to Chapter 8 — Neuropathic pain for changes that happen at each level).

In phantom pain, the supraspinal mechanism includes somatosensory cortical reorganisation of the area representing the amputated limb. Peripheral and spinal mechanisms play an important role in stump neuropathic pain.

Nociceptive pain can be due to abnormal stump tissue such as sharp bone, a weak muscle or adhesive scar. Occasionally, back conditions (e.g. from the facet or sacroiliac joints) can cause referred pain in the stump.

Assessment

History

- Site — phantom pain is an unpleasant sensation in the distribution of the lost body part. Stump pain or 'residual limb pain' is localised to the remaining body part after amputation.
- Onset — phantom pain typically starts within 6 months after the amputation and can last for many years. Stump neuropathic pain typically starts during the immediate postoperative period. Musculoskeletal pain starts with an increase in mobility.

- Character — phantom pain varies in character from neuropathic qualities such as sharp, shooting, or electric shock, to more nociceptive qualities such as dull, squeezing, aching and cramping. Stump pain is typically described as a sharp, burning, electric shock, or hypersensitive scar which can be superficial or deep in the residual limb.
- Radiation — primary pain in the stump with secondary musculoskeletal pain in the back; primary pain in the back (due to discs, facets or sacroiliac joints) with referred pain in the stump.
- Associated symptoms.
- Time/duration — continuous/intermittent.
- Exacerbating/relieving factors.
- Severity — in mixed pain conditions, commonly, the neuropathic pain component is described as the most severe.

Examination

- Inspection — skin discolouration/oedema (suggestive of infection), muscle wasting, biomechanical changes following amputation (gait, use of prosthesis, crutches).
- Palpation — Tinel's sign for scar neuroma (tapping on the injured nerve/neuroma elicits neuropathic pain); sensory examination for allodynia and hyperalgesia; examination of the back to identify referred/radicular pain originating from the spine.

Investigations

- Post-amputation pain is predominantly a clinical diagnosis based on history and examination.
- Blood tests if a chronic infection/inflammation is suspected.
- Imaging studies if structural changes are suspected.
- MRI scan of the back if radicular/referred pain from the spine is suspected.
- Quantitative sensory testing for neuropathic pain (mostly used by researchers).

Management

Management is multimodal and multidisciplinary, with a biopsychosocial approach. The objectives are symptom relief and functional restoration. The multitude of pathophysiological mechanisms mean that management has to be individually tailored.

Treatment modalities include:

- Physical therapy.
- Pharmacotherapy.
- Injection therapy.
- Neuromodulation.
- Psychological interventions.
- Surgery.

Mechanism-based treatments

Peripheral

- NSAIDs (musculoskeletal pain), lidocaine patch, capsaicin patch, menthol gel.
- Local injections (local anaesthetic nerve blocks, botulinum toxin).
- Pulsed radiofrequency treatment.
- Peripheral electrodes (neuromodulation).
- Surgery (stump refashioning, burying neuroma, reconstruction surgeries).

Spinal

- Opioids, NMDA receptor antagonists (e.g. magnesium, ketamine), sodium channel blockers (lidocaine), anticonvulsants, antidepressants.
- Spinal cord stimulation (neuromodulation).

Supraspinal

- Opioids, anticonvulsants, antidepressants.
- Cognitive behavioural therapy, biofeedback (psychological interventions).
- Mirror therapy (a simple non-invasive intervention; a mirror is placed adjacent to the normal limb to give the impression that the amputated limb is present and can be purposefully moved).
- Deep brain stimulation (neuromodulation).

Key Points

- Post-amputation pain can be described in: (i) the part of the limb that is missing; (ii) the stump; (iii) elsewhere due to biomechanical changes.
- The pain can be nociceptive or neuropathic.
- Assessment includes a history, an examination and investigations.
- Management is multimodal, directed at peripheral, spinal or supraspinal mechanisms.
- The goal is symptom relief and functional rehabilitation.

References

1. Hsu E, Cohen SP. Postamputation pain: epidemiology, mechanisms, and treatment. *J Pain Res* 2013; 6: 121.

Chapter 17

Pain in sickle cell disease

Pradeep Mukund Ingle

Sickle cell disease is a serious condition affecting red blood cells (RBCs) in the circulatory system. It is a lifelong condition which limits the life span of an individual (<50 years in most cases) suffering from it. It is more common in Afro-Caribbean and some groups of middle-eastern and south Asian populations compared with other populations.

Aetiopathology

Normal haemoglobin (Hb A) has 2α and 2β chains. Sickle cell disease is an inherited haemoglobinopathy arising due to the mutation in chromosome 11 which results in substitution of the amino acid valine for glutamate at position 6 of the β chain of haemoglobin A. This altered haemoglobin is called haemoglobin S (HB S), which is significantly unstable compared with Hb A as it loses its shape and precipitates on deoxygenation. This impacts the flexibility of RBCs along with damage to its cell membrane which then sticks to the walls of small blood vessels. This precipitation changes the shape of the red cells into a 'sickle' shape which eventually blocks the small capillaries reducing the blood flow distally causing sickle cell disease manifestations.

Depending on the proportion of Hb S, sickle cell disease can be classed into:

- Heterozygous state (sickle cell trait) — about 30 to 40% of Hb S with the rest being predominantly Hb A; usually patients are asymptomatic except under extreme physiological challenges.

- Homozygous state — characterised by almost 100% haemoglobin being Hb S. The sickling process in RBCs is much more prominent here and this can lead to occlusion of the small blood vessels (vaso-occlusive crisis) with resultant pain and a progression towards organ dysfunction leading to early death. Dehydration, abrupt temperature changes (e.g. sudden exposure to cold), physical overexertion, emotional stress, and infection can all precipitate the sickling process.

Clinical presentation

The clinical manifestations are related to the following processes that happen in sickle cell disease:

- Painful episodes — often recurrent and severe but varying in frequency from once a year to once a week.
- Anaemia — chronic anaemia which can acutely worsen in the presence of viral infections and an associated sickle cell crisis.
- Organ damage — this is a gradual process resulting from repeated physiological insults of ischaemia, infarction and inflammation affecting multiple systems. This can lead to spleen infarction and dysfunction, visual disturbance and loss of vision, renal dysfunction, pulmonary infarction and pulmonary hypertension, cardiomegaly, bone marrow failure and other musculoskeletal features such as leg ulcers. Acute strokes and TIAs can occur as a part of this process.
- Prone to infections — such as meningitis, pneumonia (e.g. *Haemophilus influenzae*, pneumococcal), cholecystitis, osteomyelitis.

Sickle cell disease patients may have various clinical features related to acute and chronic pain outlined below.

Acute painful episodes

Various presentations include typical pain episodes at the sites of long bones, ribs and the back. Note that 20% of patients may not experience these acute pains. Depending on the organs involved, these acute pain episodes can be variable in their presentations as described below:

- Acute lung syndrome — cough, haemoptysis, breathlessness, fever and resultant severe chest pain.
- Chest pain — secondary to pulmonary infarction and pleuritic in nature. Recurrent episodes can compromise lung function significantly causing eventual respiratory failure.
- Abdominal pain — secondary to various causes such as gallstones, splenic infarction, renal ischaemia, girdle syndrome (acute abdominal pain secondary to occlusion of mesenteric vessels).
- Leg pain — secondary to leg ulcers or sores.
- Pain arising from bone (long bones of extremities) and joints, mainly the hip and shoulders.
- Dactylitis/hand foot syndrome in babies due to occlusion of small capillaries by sickle-shaped RBCs.
- Priapism — painful and persistent penile erection lasting for several hours.

Chronic pain

Patients with sickle cell disease frequently suffer from chronic pain as a result of activation of central and peripheral pain signalling pathways secondary to ischaemia, infarction and inflammation processes at various sites. Associated anxiety, depression and other psychological issues arising early on in life act as barriers for optimal management of chronic pain. Chronic pain affects more than 50% of patients with sickle cell disease. Commonly, chronic pain affects the extremities, back and joints such as hips and shoulders, thereby limiting the activities and QOL from the early years. They can display features of neuropathic pain such as allodynia and hyperalgesia. Although opioids are not recommended for managing chronic pain, these patients can be put on opioids for the short term initially which can be unwittingly continued in the long term, thereby making the subsequent weaning process particularly difficult.

Investigations

- Peripheral smear — elevated reticulocyte count with evidence of sickling of RBCs.
- Sickledex test — detects the presence of Hb S (levels >10%), but it does not differentiate between a sickle cell trait and sickle cell disease. Hence, it is useful only as a screening tool, e.g. screening in pregnancy.
- Haemoglobin electrophoresis — diagnostic for sickle cell disease. It detects the percentages of each type of haemoglobin.

Management

Management is multidisciplinary with a team comprising a haematologist, paediatrician (in relevant populations), pain specialist, physiotherapist, occupational therapist, psychologist and specialist nurses. Patient education forms a vital part of preventing a painful crisis. It is important to follow local protocols for pain management in this group of patients.

The key is to prevent a vaso-occlusive crisis and precipitation of anaemia by minimising the sickling process in RBCs. This can be done by measures such as good hydration along with a healthy diet, preventing hypothermia (e.g. avoiding swimming in cold water), maintaining a warm temperature, moderate regular exercise to keep fit (but avoiding overexertion), preventing stasis (e.g. avoiding a tourniquet) and preventing infections. Acidosis and hypoxia should be avoided to minimise the chances of worsening. If an acute crisis is left untreated, it can be fatal.

Although the majority of painful episodes can be managed at home, some may need hospitalisation especially in an acute severe sickle cell crisis. These patients may already be on opioids. Some patients who have had repeated hospitalisation in the past may have poor venous access, wherein alternative routes should be considered for immediate pain control, such as subcutaneous morphine, buccal or sublingual fentanyl or intranasal diamorphine.

If repeated boluses of opioids are needed, consider patient-controlled analgesia (PCA) along with its necessary monitoring and support to prevent excessive sedation or respiratory depression.

Multimodal analgesia can often be used with synergistic effects in pain management. Mild to moderate pain can be managed with OTC analgesics such as paracetamol, NSAIDs and weak opioids.

In cases of severe pain and in some patients with moderate pain (if simple analgesics have been tried earlier), a strong opioid (morphine, oxycodone, fentanyl, etc.) may be needed.

Caution must be used with opioids in sickle cell disease. Patients with end organ damage, including renal and hepatic, can be more sensitive to the adverse effects of opioids and hence are likely to need lower doses, whereas in patients with chronic pain, who are already on long-term opioid treatment, opioid tolerance is likely to be a hurdle in pain management and increased doses may be needed.

Analgesia should be provided with sustained-release preparations of opioids for background pain, along with a provision for immediate-release opioids for breakthrough pain.

Nitrous oxide (Entonox®) can be useful in acute painful episodes in emergency departments.

Other important facets of management in sickle cell pain situations are:

- Oxygen supplementation — aim for an O$_2$ saturation of >95% to minimise the sickling process in RBCs.
- Appropriate monitoring and management of complications such as infections, stroke, osteomyelitis or an aplastic crisis.
- Psychological and social support need to be addressed similar to other long-term pain conditions. Cognitive behavioural therapy can be provided from a psychology point of view to aid the self-management of the patient's condition and long-term pain.
- Optimising the self-management of pain with improved coping mechanisms along with relaxation techniques, distraction

techniques and peer support, local heat application, TENS, and massage can all be used with varying success.

- Emergencies such as an acute chest syndrome are best managed with oxygen supplementation, analgesics, IV fluids, blood transfusions and appropriate antibiotics along with pain management as described above.
- Chronic pain may need management with tricyclic antidepressants and gabapentinoids depending on the nature of the pain.
- Antiemetics and antipruritic medications need to be used for those experiencing adverse effects with other medications.
- Regular recommended vaccinations to prevent infections, e.g. pneumococcal vaccine.
- Repeated blood transfusions or even exchange transfusions in a deteriorating patient to replace sickle cells temporarily can be beneficial in an acute painful crisis apart from their role in managing anaemia.

Stem cell transplants, although curative, carry several risks including graft versus host disease, which can have serious implications including a high mortality.

Key Points

- Sickle cell disease is a serious condition affecting RBCs which make them prone to sickling, resulting in occlusion in the small blood vessels causing a painful crisis.
- It can affect multiple body systems leading to end organ damage over a period of time resulting in an overall reduced life expectancy.
- Multidisciplinary team management, along with patient education and measures to prevent sickle cell crisis states (vaso-occlusive crisis), is the key to optimal pain management.

References

1. Wilson M, Forsyth P, Whiteside J. Haemoglobinopathy and sickle cell disease. *Contin Educ Anaesth Critical Care Pain* 2010; 10(1): 24-8.

2. https://www.nhs.uk/conditions/sickle-cell-disease/.

3. Sickle cell disease: managing acute painful episodes in hospital. NICE clinical guideline, CG143. London: National Institute for Health and Care Excellence, 2012. https://www.nice.org.uk/guidance/cg143. Accessed on 6th July 2020.

4. https://portal.e-lfh.org.uk/LearningContent/Launch/477204.

5. https://www.clinicalguidelines.scot.nhs.uk/ggc-paediatric-guidelines/ggc-guidelines/emergency-medicine/pain-in-children-management-in-the-ed/.

Chapter 18

Visceral pain

Mahesh Kodivalasa

Visceral nociceptors are sparsely spread and are predominantly made up of modified terminal ends of afferent C fibres. The autonomic nervous system acts as the main afferent conduit pathway for unmyelinated C fibres. Local tissue injury, infection and release of inflammatory mediators sensitize silent nociceptors and stimulate afferent fibres. Visceral pain is also triggered by stimuli such as smooth muscle distension or contraction, stretching of the capsule, ischaemia, necrosis, etc.

First order visceral and somatic afferent fibres converge onto the spinal cord. Convergence of both the visceral inputs and somatic inputs (from elsewhere) at the same spinal cord level — viscerosomatic convergence — explains the reason for referred pain (e.g. left arm pain with myocardial infarction).

Second order ascending pathways include the spinothalamic and also the spinoreticular pathways contributing to the emotional and autonomic components of visceral pain (e.g. a sense of impending doom along with autonomic features such as sweating and nausea with myocardial infarction).

Visceral input has a very small representation in the sensory homunculus. This in addition to the fact that the main primary ascending pathways are made of C fibres accounts for the poorly localized dull visceral pain.

Central sensitization and neuroplastic changes account for the maintenance of a chronic visceral pain status.

Red flags to consider when evaluating visceral pain include syncope, concomitant chest or back pain, breathlessness, tachycardia/palpitations, gastrointestinal or vaginal bleeding, fever, vomiting, altered or reduced bowel movements, and haemodynamic instability.

The diagnosis of functional chronic visceral pain is considered when a somatic cause cannot be found after investigations.

Management of visceral chronic abdominal pain

- A multidisciplinary approach along with patient education and psychological support is the mainstay of management.
- Medical management is based on the WHO pain ladder.
- Narcotic-induced bowel dysfunction is a real risk with opioids.
- Anti-neuropathic drugs reduce opioid requirements (high level of evidence).
- Enzyme replacement has weak evidence in chronic pancreatitis pain management.
- Interventional management aimed at blocking autonomic pathways can be tried in patients with a poor response or intolerable side effects to medical management (e.g. coeliac plexus/splanchnic nerve blocks).
- Advanced interventional management options such as spinal cord stimulation has weak evidence.
- Complementary therapies have poor evidence but can be a tool in the multimodal management package.

Management of functional chronic abdominal pain

- Patient education and reassurance are the mainstay of management (strong evidence).
- Psychological coping strategies are beneficial in the long term.
- Diet change has weak evidence.
- Probiotics have some evidence in irritable bowel disease.
- Symptomatic management may include acid prophylaxis, anti-spasmodics, laxatives, etc.

Key Points

- Viscerosomatic convergence explains the cause of the referred nature of visceral pain.
- Central sensitization and neuroplasticity explains the persistence of chronic visceral pain.

References

1. Niraj G. Pathophysiology and management of abdominal myofascial pain syndrome (AMPS): a three-year prospective audit of a management pathway in 120 patients. *Pain Medicine* 2018; 19(11): 2256-66.

2. Niraj G, Kodivalasa M, Alva S. Misdiagnosing abdominal myofascial pain syndrome (AMPS) as anterior cutaneous nerve entrapment syndrome (ACNES): are we failing patients with non-specific abdominal pain? *Interventional Pain Management Reports* 2019; 3(3): 91-7.

Chapter 19

Facial pain

Mahesh Kodivalasa

The diagnosis of facial pain depends on a good knowledge of anatomy of the nerves innervating the face. Pathology in the trigeminal nerve and cervical plexus are the predominant causes.

Trigeminal neuralgia

Trigeminal neuralgia is one of the most common craniofacial neuralgic pain conditions. The incidence is higher in women with a ratio of women > men = 2:1 (the incidence is more common above 50 years of age). The definition of trigeminal neuralgia from the IASP is: "A sudden, unilateral, severe, brief, stabbing recurrent pain in the distribution of one or more branches of the fifth cranial nerve."

Trigeminal neuralgia is typically precipitated by light touch or temperature changes in sensitive areas of the face. Maxillary and mandibular nerve dermatomes are the areas that are commonly affected.

Anatomy of the trigeminal nerve

The trigeminal nerve arises from the pons and enters Meckel's cave where the Gasserian (trigeminal) ganglion is located. The ganglion divides into ophthalmic, maxillary and mandibular nerves.

The ophthalmic nerve exits the cranium through the superior orbital fissure and innervates the skin above the eye, globe and forehead up to the vortex on the ipsilateral side.

The maxillary nerve exits the cranium through the foramen rotundum and supplies the skin between the eye and mouth on the ipsilateral side.

The mandibular nerve exits through the foramen ovale and supplies sensory innervation to the skin of the lateral part of the head, jaw, tongue and mucosa of the oral cavity. Motor fibres innervate the muscles of mastication.

Pathological mechanism/hypothesis of trigeminal neuralgia

The main proposed hypothesis is compression of the trigeminal nerve by vasculature at the dorsal root entry zone to the pons. The non-vascular compression hypothesis proposes a possible compression of the trigeminal nerve elsewhere in the path.

Aetiopathology

Peripheral sensitization of the trigeminal nerve is mainly demyelination mediated. Demyelination leads to ephaptic transmission, ectopic activity and hyperexcitability in the trigeminal nerve.

Central sensitization creates a chronic pain state by increasing excitability of the nerve and decreasing pain inhibition.

Classification and terminologies

Aetiology-based classification

Primary

- Classic (with neurovascular compression and associated morphological changes).
- Idiopathic (without neurovascular compression or neurovascular compression without morphological changes).

Secondary (symptomatic)

- Due to diseases such as tumours, multiple sclerosis, etc.

Symptom-based classification

- Typical or TN1 — intermittent intense lancinating pain for brief moments
- Atypical or TN2 — constant pain at the baseline/background.

Management

- The diagnosis of trigeminal neuralgia is mainly based on typical symptoms and signs.
- An MRI scan of the head is needed to rule out vascular compression or secondary causes.
- Red flags are: onset <40 years age, bilateral symptoms, deafness or balance issues, symptoms in other cranial nerve distributions, a cancer history, a family history of multiple sclerosis.
- Management comprises a multidisciplinary approach.
- Carbamazepine is the first-line drug for long-term management. Oxcarbazepine is an effective alternative.
- Second-line drugs include lamotrigine, gabapentinoids, amitriptyline, botulinum toxin A, baclofen and phenytoin.
- Surgical or interventional options include non-destructive (microvascular decompression — the gold standard) and destructive procedures. Surgical treatments can be helpful if pain is poorly controlled or medical treatment is poorly tolerated by the patient.
- Psychological support is recommended. Complementary therapies have very little evidence of efficacy.

Key Points

- Trigeminal neuralgia — sudden, unilateral, severe, brief, stabbing recurrent pain in the distribution of one or more branches of the fifth cranial nerve.

- Anatomy of the cranial Vth nerve — Meckel's cave, Gasserian ganglion, V1— superior orbital fissure, V2 — foramen rotundum, V3 — foramen ovale.

- Primary trigeminal neuralgia can be classic (with compression) or idiopathic (without compression); secondary trigeminal neuralgia can be due to tumours or multiple sclerosis.

- Carbamazepine is the first-line medication for trigeminal neuralgia.

References

1. Bendtsen L, Zakrzewska JM, Abbott J. European Academy of Neurology guideline on trigeminal neuralgia. *Eur J Neurol* 2020; 26: 831-49.

Chapter 20

Headaches

Mahesh Kodivalasa

The diagnosis of type of headache aids in the management and consequent success. The current widely used classification for headache is by the International Headache Society (International Classification of Headache Disorders — ICHD-3) — see ■ Table 20.1.

Table 20.1. The International Classification of Headache Disorders — ICHD-3.

Primary headaches	• Migraine. • Tension-type headache. • Trigeminal autonomic cephalalgias. • Other primary headache disorders, e.g. primary exercise headache, primary cough headache, cold stimulus headache, new daily persistent headache, etc.
Secondary headaches	• Headache attributed to head and/or neck trauma. • Headache attributed to cranial or cervical or vascular disorder. • Headache attributed to a non-vascular intracranial disorder. • Headache attributed to infection. • Headache attributed to a disorder of homeostasis. • Headache attributed to a psychiatric disorder. • Headache attributed to the cranium, neck, eyes, ears, nose, sinuses, teeth, mouth, other facial or cranial structures.

Red flags include: a sudden severe headache, headache with focal neurology, headache associated with seizures, headache associated with systemic illness, headache with neck stiffness, new onset of headache in a 50-year-old and above, change in character or pattern of headaches, history of cancer or immunosuppression, postural headache, headache that wakes from sleep and headache on waking up.

Migraine

Diagnosis based on the ICHD-3 criteria

Migraine without aura

- A. At least five headache attacks fulfilling criteria B to D (given below).
- B. Headache attacks lasting 4-72hr (untreated or unsuccessfully treated).
- C. Headache has at least two of the following four characteristics:
  - unilateral location;
  - pulsating quality;
  - moderate or severe pain intensity;
  - aggravation by or causing avoidance of routine physical activity (e.g. walking or climbing stairs).
- D. During headache at least one of the following:
  - nausea and/or vomiting;
  - photophobia and phonophobia.
- Not better accounted for by another ICHD-3 diagnosis.

Migraine with aura

- A. At least two attacks fulfilling criteria B and C.
- B. One or more of the following fully reversible aura symptoms:
  - visual;
  - sensory;
  - speech and/or language.
- C. At least two of the following four characteristics:
  - at least one aura symptom spreads gradually over 5 minutes;

- two or more aura symptoms occur in succession;
- each individual aura symptom lasts 5-60 minutes;
- at least one aura symptom is unilateral;
- at least one aura symptom is positive;
- the aura is accompanied, or followed within 60 minutes, by headache.
- D. Not better accounted for by another ICHD-3 diagnosis.

Typical phases of migraine

The typical phases of a migraine include the prodromal phase (premonitory symptoms), headache (with or without preceding aura) and postdromal phase.

Pathophysiology of migraine

The proposed mechanism for migraine includes activation of the trigemino-vascular system, sensitization and changes in central modulation.

Treatment of migraine

Abortive treatment

- A step-ladder approach may be used, initiating with an analgesic (NSAID) along with an antiemetic and then escalating to a 5-HT1 receptor agonist (triptan) along with an antiemetic or vice versa. Paracetamol may also be tried concomitantly. Altering the agents and route of administration can be beneficial.
- The endpoint is a reduction in severity within 2 hours.
- Abortive treatment for more than 8 days in a month is shown to be associated with medication overuse and analgesic rebound headaches. This is shown to be mostly associated with opioids, barbiturates, ergotamine and caffeine preparations.

Preventive treatment

- Indicated if the frequency of migraines is more than four per month.
- First line — topiramate, propranolol.
- Second line — tricyclic antidepressants (amitriptyline), serotonin-norepinephrine reuptake inhibitor (duloxetine).
- Acupuncture may also help as a complementary therapy.
- Third line — botulinum injections (PREEMPT 1 and 2 trials) — NICE recommends this in patients with a frequency of migraines more than eight per month and who have tried three different preventive medicines.
- A good response to preventative treatment is considered as a reduction in headache severity and frequency by 50%.
- Other interventional options include: greater occipital nerve block, occipital nerve stimulation, transcutaneous electrical stimulation of the supraorbital nerve, transcutaneous stimulation of the cervical branch of the vagus nerve, etc.

Key Points

- Headaches can be primary or secondary (ICHD-3 classification).
- Red flags have to be ruled out.
- Migraine without aura — at least five headaches along with other diagnostic criteria.
- Migraine with aura — at least two headaches along with other diagnostic criteria.
- Abortive treatment — NSAIDs or triptans with an antiemetic.
- Preventive treatment — first line — topiramate, propranolol; second line — amitriptyline, SNRI, acupuncture; third line — Botox®.

References

1.   Headache Classification Committee of the International Headache Society (IHS). The International Classification of Headache Disorders, 3rd edition. *Cephalalgia* 2018; 38(1): 1-211.

2.   Botulinum toxin type A for the prevention of headaches in adults with chronic migraine. NICE Technology appraisal guidance, TA260. London: National Institute for Health and Care Excellence, 2012. https://www.nice.org.uk/guidance/ta260. Accessed on 7th July 2020.

Chapter 21

Pelvic pain

Mahesh Kodivalasa

Chronic pelvic pain is a persistent pain associated with pelvic contents including gastrointestinal, genitourinary, pelvic floor musculoskeletal and neural structures.

Knowing the source and the type of pain (e.g. visceral, somatic, neuropathic and mixed) can aid in the management. Pelvic cancer pain is predominantly a mixed type of pain.

Chronic pelvic pain is one of the conditions associated with a significant psychosocial impact.

Classification of pelvic pain by the European Association of Urology uses a system which not only accounts for the source of pain, but also the type of pain and the psychosocial impact.

Aetiopathology

Triggering events such as trauma, infection and inflammation stimulate nociceptors. An intense primary stimulus or repetitive stimuli lead to sensitization and recruitment of silent nociceptors.

Chronic pelvic pain is more prevalent in women than in men. Inflammatory causes are commoner in females while traumatic (including post-surgical) causes are associated with the majority of cases in men.

Central sensitization (and receptor field expansion) lead to the maintenance of a chronic pelvic pain status.

Viscerosomatic convergence is responsible for the referred pain experienced by patients.

Management

- The management of chronic pelvic pain involves a coordinated multidisciplinary approach.
- An effective management of chronic pelvic pain begins with a thorough history including symptomatology to understand the source and trigger. It is essential to explore psychosocial factors and their impact.
- The history should include information about the associated organ systems (e.g. gastrointestinal — altered bowel habits; genitourinary — cyclical pain, dyspareunia, dysuria; musculoskeletal and neurological — postural variability).
- Medical management is mainly based on the WHO ladder starting with simple analgesics.
- Anti-neuropathic medications are particularly helpful in pelvic pain with neuropathic features. Side effects of some drugs such as amitriptyline (urinary retention) may be beneficial.
- Hormonal therapy may be tried in patients with cyclical pain.
- Topical therapies with local anaesthetic creams, gels and patches can help.
- A thorough knowledge of somatic innervation of pelvic structures helps in directing targeted interventional management appropriately.
- Interventional management options range from simple to complex procedures.
- Peripheral nerve injections like pudendal nerve, ilio-inguinal, ilio-hypogastric and genitofemoral blocks inhibit the ascending inputs.
- Interventions aiming at autonomic pathways are mainly performed for visceral pain (including cancer pathology). The ganglion of impar and superior hypogastric plexus are the main targets.

- Intrathecal neurolysis is an intervention that is particularly helpful in patients with terminal pelvic cancer, a limited life span and intractable pain or intolerable side effects with medical management.
- Neuromodulation is shown to be helpful in carefully selected cases.
- Pelvic floor exercises, relaxation techniques, complementary therapy (TENS, acupuncture) and psychological interventions are all part of a multidisciplinary approach.

Key Points

- Pelvic pain can be visceral, somatic, neuropathic or mixed.
- Chronic pelvic pain has a significant psychosocial impact.
- Viscerosomatic convergence can explain referral patterns.
- Gastrointestinal, genitourinary, musculoskeletal and neurological features should be considered during assessment and management.
- Injections can aim at either peripheral nerves or at the autonomic plexuses, in addition to centroneuraxial blocks.

References

1. https://uroweb.org/guideline/chronic-pelvic-pain/.
2. Cottrell AM, Schneider MP, Goonewardene S, *et al*. Benefits and harms of electrical neuromodulation for chronic pelvic pain: a systematic review. *Eur Urol Focus* 2020; 6(3): 559-71.

Chapter 22

Cancer pain

Mahesh Kodivalasa

30-50% of patients with cancer can experience moderate to severe pain during the course of cancer illness. 30% of patients with cancer are at risk of poor pain control especially in their last year. 75-95% of patients with metastatic or advanced cancer suffer with severe pain.

Cancer pain often does not fit into a single pain state: pain can be nociceptive (50%), neuropathic (10%) or mixed (40%).

Aetiology or mechanisms of cancer pain

- As a direct result of the disease — rapidly growing encapsulated tumours, ischaemic necrosis of the tumour itself, bone metastasis, compression of surrounding structures, bowel occlusion, raised intracranial pressure, etc.
- General effects from the illness — painful pressure areas, chronic illness neuropathy and myopathy.
- Treatment-related — chemotherapy- and radiotherapy-related neuropathic pain, chronic post-surgical pain, etc.
- Unrelated causes — pre-existing pain (e.g. arthritis and other chronic pain conditions).

Mechanisms of bone pain in cancer

- Metastatic lesions lead to stretching of the periosteum and radicular pain from compression of bone tissue, surrounding structures and nerves.

- Fractures secondary to osteoclastic activity.
- Osteclastic activity induced chemolysis and local acidosis sensitize and stimulate nociceptors.

Total pain from cancer includes a constant background pain and breakthrough pain. The management plan should include anticipation and prescription for breakthrough pain.

Management

- History — remember the acronym SOCRATES (see Chapter 2). The assessment of physical, psychological and social impact, drug history and past medical history should be part of the cancer pain evaluation.
- Examination to aid diagnosis of neuropathic vs. nociceptive vs. mixed pain.
- Relevant investigations — especially if interventional management is planned in patients undergoing chemoradiotherapy.
- A pain management plan should include a multidisciplinary pharmacological and non-pharmacological approach.
- Pain complaints may change over the course of cancer illness and correspondingly analgesic requirements too. Interdisciplinary communication aids in understanding the disease progress and prognosis. Poor pain management has a devastating psychological and social impact on patients and their families.
- A robust cancer pain management plan should be flexible for adequate pain control and tailored for a meaningful social quality of life for the patient.

Pharmacological cancer pain management

- Medications are mainly based on the WHO ladder:
  - by the clock — regular doses rather than by demand;
  - by the mouth — for ease of administration; and
  - by the ladder — effective minimal dose with tolerable side effects for the patient.
- Short-acting opioid drugs in addition to helping with titration of medications also aid in the management of unstable and breakthrough pain.

- Long-acting agents are more suitable for the management of stable pain.
- The management of cancer pain with opioids may need opioid rotation or switching if the patient develops tolerance or intolerable side effects.
- Commonly used adjuvant drugs include paracetamol, NSAIDs and anti-neuropathic pain medications.
- Other useful adjuvant drugs in cancer pain management include:
  - corticosteroids — bone pain, cerebral metastasis and tumour oedema;
  - antispasmodics and muscle relaxants — smooth muscle and skeletal muscle spasms;
  - bisphosphonates — bone pain.

Non-interventional and non-pharmacological cancer pain management

- Education.
- Psychotherapy.
- Physiotherapy.
- Complementary therapy — TENS, acupuncture, massage, aromatherapy, etc.

Other multidisciplinary management options

- Oncological — chemoradiotherapy.
- Surgical — curative/palliative/debulking procedures.
- Hormonal therapy.

Interventional cancer pain management procedures

Main indications

- Persistence of pain despite pharmacological management (up to 10% of patients on the WHO ladder experience ongoing significant pain).
- Intolerable side effects with conventional therapy.
- A need for rapid analgesia (severe pain and or short life expectancy).

- Pain responsive to blocks (confined somatic pain, visceral pain, etc).

Types of interventions

- Simple non-destructive procedures — e.g. trigger point injections, peripheral nerve blocks, neuromodulation, systemic infusion techniques, peri-neural and central neuraxial infusion techniques.
- Destructive procedures (mainly in patients with limited life expectancy) — neurolytic blocks (e.g. coeliac plexus block), radiofrequency ablation, surgery (e.g. myelotomy), intrathecal neurolysis, cordotomy, etc.

Key Points

- Cancer pain can be nociceptive (50%), neuropathic (10%) or mixed (40%).
- The WHO pain ladder: by the clock, by the mouth and by the ladder.
- Management is with interdisciplinary communication and multimodal pain management.
- Pharmacological, non-pharmacological, multidisciplinary intervention, injection therapies and psychological support can be utilised.

References

1. Bennett MI. Mechanism-based cancer-pain therapy. *Pain* 2017; 158 Suppl 1: S74-8.
2. Paice JA, Mulvey M, Bennett M, *et al.* AAPT diagnostic criteria for chronic cancer pain conditions. *J Pain* 2017; 18(3): 233-46.
3. Falk S, Dickenson AH. Pain and nociception: mechanisms of cancer-induced bone pain. *J Clin Oncol* 2014; 32(16): 1647-54.
4. Scott-Warren J, Bhaskar A. Cancer pain management — part I: general principles. *Contin Educ Anaesth Crit Care Pain* 2014; 14(6): 278-84.
5. Scott-Warren J, Bhaskar A. Cancer pain management — part II: interventional techniques. *Contin Educ Anaesth Crit Care Pain* 2015; 15(2): 68-72.

Chapter 23

Injection therapy for chronic pain — nerve blocks

Shyam Balasubramanian

Indications

Nerve blocks for chronic pain management can be for diagnostic or therapeutic indications. The procedures can be temporary (local anaesthesia +/- steroids) or permanent (chemical or physical neurolysis).

Nerve blocks are indicated for musculoskeletal pain (e.g. suprascapular nerve block for shoulder pain) as well as neuropathic pain (e.g. inguinal nerve block for persistent post-hernia repair neuropathic pain).

Benefits

Injection therapies are one aspect of multimodal intervention in managing chronic pain. Injections are performed for symptom relief as well as to help patients engage with functional rehabilitation.

Types of nerve blocks

Nerves can be blocked at different levels:

- Axial — spinal, epidural.
- Paraxial — paravertebral, erector spinae plane, plexus blocks.
- Peripheral — e.g. upper and lower limb nerve blocks, trunk blocks.

Medications injected

- Local anaesthetics — lidocaine, bupivacaine, levobupivacaine. These act by blocking the sodium channels in the neurons. In a cohort of patients with chronic pain, the duration of pain relief outlasts the duration of action of the local anaesthetics. An explanation for this extended pain relief includes interrupting the vicious cycle of pain → spasm → more pain.
- Steroids — despite limited evidence, steroids such as depo-methylprednisolone, triamcinolone, dexamethasone are used in nerve blocks. The proposed mechanism of action includes membrane stabilisation, an anti-inflammatory effect and a local effect.

Complications of nerve blocks

Generic complications include: infection, bleeding/bruising, allergy/anaphylaxis, injection soreness/exacerbation of pain.

Trauma can occur due to the needle used — nerve injury, vascular injury — depending on the anatomical location of the injection (pneumothorax, visceral injuries, etc).

There are also risks due to the medications used:

- Generic — local anaesthetic toxicity, systemic and local effects of steroids.
- Medication deposited in the right site, but still producing unwanted effects — e.g. Horner's syndrome following a stellate ganglion block, hypotension following epidural injections, sensory/motor blockade following peripheral nerve blocks.
- Medication deposited in the wrong site — e.g. accidental intravascular injections, accidental epidural/intrathecal injections.

Key Points

- Nerve blocks are offered for diagnostic or therapeutic indications.
- Nerve blocks can be temporary or permanent.
- Permanent blocks can be conducted by chemical or physical means.
- Nerves are blocked at the axial, paraxial or peripheral levels.
- Risks can be generic, due to the needle, or due to the medications used.

References

1. Tumber PS, Peng PW. Peripheral nerve blocks in chronic pain. In: *Multimodality imaging guidance in interventional pain management*. Narouze SN, Ed. Oxford University Press, 2016: 441.

2. Manchikanti L, Kaye AD, Falco FJ, Hirsch JA, Eds. *Essentials of interventional techniques in managing chronic pain*. Springer, 2018.

Chapter 24

Injection therapy for chronic pain — facet interventions

Thanthullu Vasu

Facet medial nerve block injections are one of the most common injections performed in a pain service for spinal pain. Lumbar facet pain accounts for 10-15% of low back pain. Diagnostic nerve blocks followed by radiofrequency denervation has a high level of evidence for their use; they are recommended by NICE guidelines for low back pain if non-surgical modalities do not help (recommendation 1.3.2, NG59). Cervical and thoracic medial nerve blocks are less commonly performed than the lumbar blocks.

Facet joints are formed by the articulation of the inferior articular process of the vertebra above with the superior articular process of the lower vertebra. They are covered by synovial cartilage which is richly innervated.

Any injection in a chronic pain service will form part of a comprehensive multimodal management including education and explanation, exercises and pacing, coping strategies to achieve functional restoration, and improvement in quality of life. Various guidelines and techniques have been published, but the clinician performing the block should be fully trained and aware of the risks of the most familiar techniques used. Any block should be conducted with due diligence for safety. Safe, aseptic precautions are vital in any spinal injection procedure.

Indications for a medial branch block:

- Localised spinal pain without radiculopathy.
- Duration of pain lasting at least 3 months.
- No response to conservative treatment including physiotherapy and medications.

Contraindications for a medial branch block:

- Active infection either systemically or locally.
- Patient refusal.
- Allergy to local anaesthetic.

X-ray imaging is used following the ALARA (as low as reasonably achievable) principle. The approach and technique depend on the training and decision of the performing clinician as well as the level at which the injection is performed.

The vertebral lower border is 'squared' to avoid a parallax error; a lateral oblique view gives the 'scotty dog' view to help correlate the anatomy.

The injection is done at the level where the pain corresponds to the transverse process; the branch from one higher level is also blocked to make sure that all the nerves supplying a particular facet joint are blocked.

Diagnostic injections are usually performed with 0.5ml of local anaesthetic. The patient is given a pain diary to record the response to the injection. It is vital to educate patients with this assessment as it helps in deciding whether radiofrequency denervation will help.

Key Points

- Lumbar facet pain accounts for 10-15% of low back pain.
- Diagnostic blocks are used for diagnostic purposes before proceeding with radiofrequency procedures.
- Due care and diligence should be taken, as for any other spinal injection procedure.
- Assessment with a pain diary is vital after the procedure.

References

1. Saravanakumar K, Harvey A. Lumbar zygapophyseal (facet) joint pain. *Rev Pain* 2008; 2(1): 8-13.

2. Low back pain and sciatica in over 16s: assessment and management. NICE guideline, NG59. London: National Institute for Health and Care Excellence, 2016. https://www.nice.org.uk/guidance/ng59. Accessed on 6th July 2020.

3. Safety practives for interventional pain procedures. Spine Intevention Society. Available at: https://www.spineintervention.org/page/Safety_Practices. Accessed on 1st May 2020.

Chapter 25

Injection therapy for chronic pain — radiofrequency procedures

Thanthullu Vasu

Radiofrequency (RF) is a non-ionising radiation, at the lower end of the electromagnetic spectrum, and includes radiowaves and microwaves. A high-frequency alternating current (in the amplitude modulation — AM band; 50 to 500kHz; low energy) is used to interrupt nociceptive pathways at various regions of the body. This current will cause molecules within the tissues to oscillate and the resulting friction between molecules release thermal energy.

Two types of radiofrequency commonly used include:

- Continuous RF — heat from a thermal lesion is used to interrupt nerve conduction. Lumbar and cervical facet medial nerves are the common sites blocked. The trigeminal ganglion can be denervated for facial pain.
- Pulsed RF — neuromodulation rather than thermal energy is the key for pulsed RF. The exact modalities including time duration and cycles are still being researched; usually 20ms pulses and 2Hz frequency are used for 2 minutes, resulting in a temperature of less than 42°C. Pulsed RF is safer than continuous if the fluoroscopic image is not clear, as the risk of motor nerve damage is less.

Lumbar facet medial nerve radiofrequency denervation

Indications:

- Positive response to a diagnostic block.
- Patient consent.
- Chronic low back pain that has not responded to conservative management.

Contraindications:

- Active infection either systemically or locally.
- Patient refusal.
- Allergy to medications or an inability to use fluoroscopy.

Lumbar facet medial nerve radiofrequency denervation has a good level of evidence for its use and is recommended by NICE guidelines (NG59) for low back pain if conservative treatment has failed.

Safety precautions including asepsis, X-ray safety and clinical governance issues should be considered with due diligence. A dispersive pad should be applied to the skin, usually on the ipsilateral thigh. The patient should be educated regarding the practicalities to achieve maximum cooperation during sensory and motor testing. Sensory testing is done with a current of 50Hz, 1ms pulse width and voltage up to 0.5v. Motor testing is done at 2Hz and 1ms pulse width, voltage tested to maximum and observed at the particular dermatome on the ipsilateral leg. Lateral X-ray views are vital before performing nerve destruction procedures. Ipsilateral oblique and lateral X-ray views with a final position of the needle should be saved for future records. 0.5ml of 1% lidocaine is injected before lesioning; then a one-minute 80°C lesion is made. It is important to denervate all the nerves that were blocked during the diagnostic block.

Key Points

- Radiofrequency denervation uses a high-frequency alternating current.
- Two types include continuous and pulsed.
- Pulsed RF uses neuromodulation rather than thermal denervation and has a safety profile with regards to a motor block.
- The actual parameters for pulsed RF are still debatable.
- Lumbar facet medial nerve RF has a high level of evidence for its use and is recommended by the NICE NG59 guidelines.

References

1. Rea W, Kapur S, Mutagi H. Radiofrequency therapies in chronic pain. *Contin Educ Anaesth Critical Care Pain* 2011; 11(2): 35-8.

2. Low back pain and sciatica in over 16s: assessment and management. NICE guideline, NG59. London: National Institute for Health and Care Excellence, 2016. https://www.nice.org.uk/guidance/ng59. Accessed on 6th July 2020.

Chapter 26

Injection therapy for chronic pain — epidural injections

Shyam Balasubramanian

Epidural injections are used in chronic pain to deposit steroids near an inflamed nerve root and other areas of inflammation in the spinal canal area. Conditions such as intervertebral disc rupture can release neuropeptides and prostaglandins which can sensitize the free nerve endings causing back pain, and sensitize the nerve roots and dorsal root ganglion causing radicular pain.

Indications

- Radicular pain (nerve root irritation).
- Spinal pain due to an inflammatory cause.
- Discogenic pain.

Epidural injections are not recommended for simple mechanical back pain. Epidural injections are not supported by NICE for spinal stenosis.

Contraindications

- Local/systemic infection.
- Altered coagulation.

Technique

Preparation is key — the 4Ps:

- Preparation of the patient (pre-procedural assessment, consent).
- Preparation of the procedure room (monitoring, access to resuscitation facilities, medications, trained assistant).
- Preparation of the site (positioning, asepsis).
- Performance of the block.

The Faculty of Pain Medicine (Royal College of Anaesthetists) recommends intravenous access and monitoring (ECG, blood pressure, pulse oximetry). Epidural injections should be done under fluoroscopy guidance after confirming the satisfactory spread of contrast.

There are three approaches (■ Figure 26.1):

- Interlaminar epidural.
- Transforaminal epidural.
- Caudal epidural.

A caudal epidural involves introducing the needle through the sacrococcygeal membrane. An interlaminar epidural involves introducing the needle between the upper and lower laminae to reach the ligamentum flava, with either a midline or paramedian approach. A transforaminal epidural has a more lateral approach — the needle is introduced into the intervertebral foramen where the nerve root (and the accompanying vessels) are located.

Medications injected

- Local anaesthetics.
- Glucocorticoids:
  - particulate — methylprednisolone, triamcinolone;
  - soluble — dexamethasone.

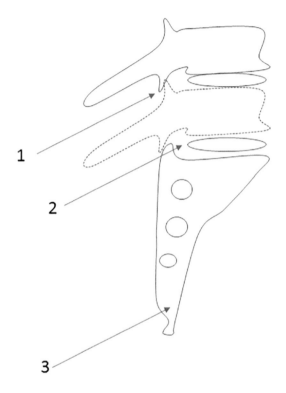

Figure 26.1. Approaches used for epidural injections: 1. Interlaminar epidural; 2. Transforaminal epidural; 3. Caudal epidural.

When administered through the transforaminal route, particulate steroids carry a risk of embolism if inadvertently injected into the artery. Hence, methylprednisolone and triamcinolone are used in the caudal and interlaminar approach, but dexamethasone is recommended for the transforaminal approach.

Comparison of techniques

The various types of epidural injections are highlighted in ■ Table 26.1.

Table 26.1. Comparison of types of epidural injections.

Caudal epidural	Interlaminar epidural	Transforaminal epidural
Familiar technique.	Familiar technique.	Requires technical expertise.
Mainly for sacral, lower lumbar radicular pain.	Used for radicular pain from any spinal level.	Used for radicular pain from any spinal level.
Non-specific; needs a higher volume to cover the desired levels.	Specific to the desired level; but still needs the volume to reach the anterior aspect of the spinal canal.	Very specific; a minimal volume is sufficient as the injectate is deposited directly around the nerve root of interest.
As the volume of the injectate is high, the actual amount of steroid around each nerve root is limited which can reduce effectiveness.	The amount of steroid reaching the specific nerve root is better than in the caudal approach.	As the steroid is directly delivered close to the nerve root, the effectiveness of this approach is potentially more.
The presence of epidural septa and scars can affect the anterior spread of the injectate (where the discs and nerve roots are located).	The presence of epidural septa and scars can affect the anterior spread of the injectate (where the discs and nerve roots are located).	A more predictable anterior spread, in particular when the injectate has to reliably reach the nerve roots.
A safer technique with a negligible risk of accidental dural puncture.	Risks include accidental dural puncture and damage to the cord.	As the needle enters the transforaminal space, there is a higher risk of damage to the nerve root and inadvertent intravascular injection.

Complications

Generic complications include: infection, bleeding/bruising, allergy/anaphylaxis, injection soreness/exacerbation of pain.

Trauma can occur due to the needle used: nerve injury (lumbar nerve roots), vascular injury, dural puncture and spinal cord injury.

There are also risks due to the medications used:

- Generic — systemic and local effects of steroids.
- Medication deposited in the correct site, but still producing unwanted effects — e.g. hypotension, bladder retention.
- Medication deposited in the wrong site — e.g. accidental intravascular injections, accidental intrathecal injections.

Please also refer to Chapter 5, Back pain and Chapter 51, Pharmacology — steroids.

Key Points

- Epidural steroid injections are indicated in radicular pain and spinal pain of inflammatory origin.
- They are not recommended for simple musculoskeletal back pain and spinal canal stenosis.
- The three approaches are caudal, interlaminar and transforaminal.
- Risks can be generic, due to the needle, or due to the medications used.

References

1.   Collighan N, Gupta S. Epidural steroids. *Contin Educ Anaesth Critical Care Pain* 2009; 10(1): 1-5.

2.   Low back pain and sciatica in over 16s: assessment and management. NICE guideline, NG59. London: National Institute for Health and Care Excellence, 2016. https://www.nice.org.uk/guidance/ng59. Accessed on 6th July 2020.

Chapter 27

Injection therapy for chronic pain — neurolytic procedures

Shyam Balasubramanian

When diagnostic injection with local anaesthetic alone produces good meaningful pain relief, then neurolytic procedures are used to prolong the benefit of these injections. A neurolytic block is the targeted destruction of neural structures to cause physical interruption of pain signals (■ Figure 27.1).

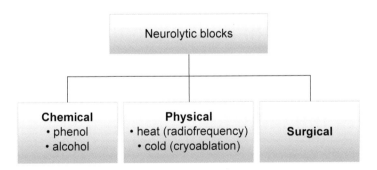

Figure 27.1. Neurolytic blocks.

Apart from a limited number of treatments (such as facet joint denervation for back/neck pain), neurolytic procedures are predominantly reserved for chronic cancer pain management. The two clinical entities, deafferentation pain and neuroma pain which can follow neurolysis after a few months, can be extremely difficult to manage. Hence, there is hesitancy in routinely offering neurolytic procedures for chronic non-cancer pain.

Examples of neurolytic blocks:

- Axial — intrathecal phenol, radiofrequency cordotomy.
- Paraxial — coeliac plexus neurolysis, lumbar sympathectomy, splanchnic nerve radiofrequency denervation, facet nerve radiofrequency denervation.
- Peripheral — intercostal nerves, inguinal nerves, etc.

Chemical neurolysis

There are two chemicals used:

- Phenol — 5-8% concentration causes non-selective destruction of the sympathetic and somatosensory nerves. Phenol denatures proteins, and so the nerve undergoes demyelination.
- Alcohol — 35-100% concentration causes non-selective destruction of the nerve fibres. Alcohol extracts lipids from the nerve tissue and causes precipitation of proteins. Alcohol is an irritant and can cause pain on injection which can be minimised by injecting with local anaesthetics.

Phenol is hyperbaric and alcohol is hypobaric when administered intrathecally. This has implications on positioning the patient after the injection (e.g. following intrathecal phenol, the painful area should be dependent). For other injections (such as coeliac plexus neurolysis) there is not much difference in clinical effectiveness between phenol and alcohol.

Physical neurolysis

Radiofrequency

The procedure involves generating current with an oscillating frequency that produces heat locally. A needle with an active tip is introduced close to the neural structure. An electrode is passed through the needle and the active tip is selectively heated with a predetermined temperature for the duration (e.g. 80°C for 90 seconds).

Cryoablation

The procedure involves percutaneous insertion of a cryoprobe and exposing the nerves to an extreme cold temperature. When compared to radiofrequency denervation, cryoablation may have a lesser risk of formation of neuroma and post-procedural hyperalgesia.

Complications of neurolytic blocks

(Refer to Chapter 23 on the complications of nerve blocks.)

Generic complications

- Trauma due to the needle.
- Risks due to the lesioning technique (chemical/physical):
  - lesion in the right site (e.g. hypotension following coeliac plexus neurolysis);
  - lesion in the wrong site (e.g. sciatic nerve root damage following facet joint radiofrequency denervation).
- Worsening of the pain:
  - deafferentation pain — follows any injury to the nervous system. Possibly because of reorganisation of the nervous system after an injury, patients can experience spontaneous pain in the parts of the body distal to the nerve injury;

- neuroma — a tangle of sensitive neural fibres and connective tissue follows nerve injury. Patients can experience hyperalgesia in the injured area and tapping over the neuroma can produce sudden burning/stabbing pain (Tinel's sign).

Key Points

- Neurolytic blocks involve destruction of neural structures.
- These blocks can be conducted by chemical or physical means.
- Nerves are permanently blocked at the axial, paraxial or peripheral levels.
- Risks can be generic, due to the needle, or due to the medications used.

References

1. Filippiadis DK, Cornelis FH, Kelekis A. Interventional oncologic procedures for pain palliation. *La Presse Médicale* 2019; 48(7-8): e251-6.

2. Plancarte R, Hernández Porras C. Interventional pain management in cancer patients. *Postgrad Med J* 2020; DOI: 10.1080/00325481.2020.1757953.

Chapter 28

Injection therapy for chronic pain — stellate ganglion block

Shyam Balasubramanian

Applied anatomy

The stellate ganglion, also called the cervicothoracic ganglion (C7, T1), is formed by the fusion of the inferior cervical and first thoracic ganglion (■ Figure 28.1). It provides sympathetic outflow to the head and upper limb. The

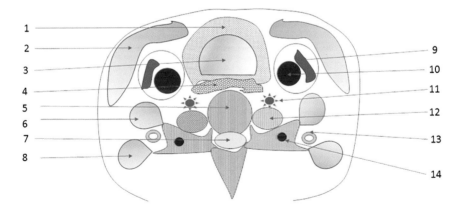

Figure 28.1. The stellate ganglion: 1. Thyroid gland; 2. Sternocleidomastoid muscle; 3. Trachea; 4. Oesophagus; 5. C6 vertebral body; 6. Scalene anterior muscle; 7. Spinal cord; 8. Scalene medius muscle; 9. Internal jugular vein; 10. Carotid artery; 11. Cervical sympathetic chain; 12. Longus colli muscle; 13. C6 nerve root; 14. Vertebral artery.

ganglion is located anterolateral to the longus colli muscle (covered by prevertebral fascia) which in turn originates from the transverse processes of C5 to T3. The ganglion is located posterior to the carotid sheath, lateral to the oesophagus/C7 vertebral body, above the apex of the lung and medial to the vertebral artery/cervical nerve roots.

The vertebral artery runs anterior to the C7 transverse process, close to the cervical sympathetic chain, but runs through the foramen transversarium from C6 upwards. Because of the vicinity to the lung and the vertebral artery, to minimise risks, a stellate ganglion block is traditionally performed at the C6 level.

Indications

- Pain indications — sympathetically mediated pain (e.g. CRPS, although not supported by NICE guidelines), neuropathic pain.
- Vascular insufficiency — arterial embolism in the upper limb, frostbite, Raynaud's disease, refractory angina.
- Miscellaneous — hyperhydrosis.

Contraindications

Relative contraindications include:

- Local infection.
- Altered coagulation.
- Recent myocardial infarction.
- Contralateral phrenic nerve palsy.

Technique

Preparation is key — the 4Ps:

- Preparation of the patient (pre-procedural assessment, consent).

- Preparation of the procedure room (monitoring, access to resuscitation facilities, medications, trained assistant).
- Preparation of the site (positioning, asepsis).
- Performance of the block.

Intravenous access and standard monitoring (ECG, blood pressure, pulse oximetry) should be in place.

The block is performed with the landmark technique, fluoroscopy guidance and under ultrasound guidance. With the patient in the supine position, Chassaignac's tubercle (anterior tubercle of C6) is palpated; carotid artery pulsation is felt. The needle is inserted between the trachea and the carotid artery with the aim to hit the transverse process of C6. The needle is withdrawn by a few millimetres so that the needle tip lies anterior to the longus colli muscle. After careful negative aspiration, the injectate is carefully deposited.

Under fluoroscopy, contrast is injected prior to the deposition of the medication. This is to rule out intravascular injection and to confirm the cephalo-cranial spread of the dye on the surface of longus colli.

Ultrasound increases the precision and safety of the procedure. The ability to visualise the soft tissues (longus colli), vascular structures (carotid artery, vertebral artery, inferior thyroid artery, internal jugular vein) and neural structures (brachial plexus nerve roots) makes an ultrasound-guided block more attractive. If during the traditional approach of inserting the needle between the trachea and carotid sheath, the inferior thyroid artery gets in the way inside the thyroid gland, ultrasound enables the option of a lateral (to the carotid sheath) to medial approach.

Under the landmark technique and fluoroscopy guidance, higher volumes (approximately 10ml) were commonly used. With ultrasound, however, precision has facilitated effective blocks with lower volumes (3-5ml).

A successful block is confirmed with the occurrence of Horner's syndrome (ptosis, miosis, anhydrosis).

Complications

Generic complications include: infection, bleeding/bruising, allergy/anaphylaxis, injection soreness/exacerbation of pain.

Trauma can occur due to the needle used: nerve injury (cervical nerve roots, phrenic nerve, vagus nerve), vascular injury (carotid, vertebral, inferior thyroid artery), pneumothorax, oesophageal/tracheal perforation, chylothorax due to thoracic duct injury.

There are also risks due to the medications used:

- Generic — local anaesthetic toxicity, systemic and local effects of steroids.
- Medication deposited in the right site, but still producing unwanted effects — e.g. Horner's syndrome, hoarseness of voice due to a recurrent laryngeal nerve block, paralysis of the hemidiaphragm due to a phrenic nerve block.
- Medication deposited in the wrong site — e.g. accidental intravascular injections, accidental epidural/intrathecal injections.

Key Points

- Cervicothoracic ganglia provide sympathetic innervation to the head, neck and upper limb.
- A stellate ganglion is blocked for pain and vascular indications.
- The vicinity to the vertebral artery and other neurovascular structures mandates extreme caution.
- The block is traditionally conducted at the C6 level.
- Risks can be generic, due to the needle, or due to the medications used.

References

1.   Piraccini E, Munakomi S, Chang KV. Stellate ganglion blocks. StatPearls [Internet], 2020. StatPearls Publishing. Available at: https://www.ncbi.nlm.nih.gov/books/NBK507798/. Accessed on 8th July 2020.

Chapter 29

Injection therapy for chronic pain — lumbar sympathetic block

Shyam Balasubramanian

Applied anatomy

The lumbar sympathetic chain runs anterolateral to the lumbar vertebral bodies L1 to L4, anterior to the psoas sheath (■ Figure 29.1). The preganglionic neurons leave the spinal cord (L1 to L4 nerve roots) through the

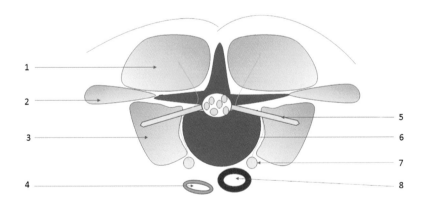

Figure 29.1. Lumbar sympathetic chain: 1. Erector spinae muscle; 2. Quadratus lumborum muscle; 3. Psoas major muscle; 4. Inferior vena cava; 5. Lumbar spinal nerve root; 6. L3 vertebral body; 7. Lumbar sympathetic chain; 8. Aorta.

white rami communicans and synapse at the corresponding lumbar sympathetic ganglion. The postganglionic neurons provide sympathetic innervation to the lower limbs. As the sympathetic chain is denser at L2/L3, commonly the block is performed at the lower aspect of the L2 or upper aspect of the L3 vertebral body.

Indications

- Pain indications — sympathetic mediated neuropathic pain in the lower limbs, CRPS (although this is not recommended in the NICE guidelines).
- Vascular indications — critical peripheral vascular disease, frostbite.
- Miscellaneous — hyperhydrosis.

Contraindications

Relative contraindications include:

- Local infection.
- Altered coagulation, etc.

Technique

Preparation is key — the 4Ps:

- Preparation of the patient (pre-procedural assessment, consent).
- Preparation of the procedure room (monitoring, access to resuscitation facilities, medications, trained assistant).
- Preparation of the site (positioning, asepsis).
- Performance of the block.

Intravenous access and standard monitoring (ECG, blood pressure, pulse oximetry) should be in place.

The block is usually carried out under fluoroscopy guidance. With the patient in the prone position, under fluoroscopy guidance, the bodies of the L2 and L3 vertebra are identified. After skin infiltration with local anaesthetic, the spinal needle is introduced lateral to medial, aiming for the anterior aspect of the vertebral body. Once the needle is in contact with the vertebral body, the fluoroscopy is positioned to show the lateral view. The anteroposterior view is for the direction and the lateral view is for depth. The tip of the needle should be 3-5mm dorsal to the anterior border of the vertebral body. The fluoroscopy is moved back to the anteroposterior view. Contrast is injected to demonstrate smooth cephalo-cranial spread, anterior to the psoas muscle.

If the sympathetic block is for diagnostic purpose, local anaesthesia +/- steroids are deposited after careful negative aspiration. If the block is for therapeutic purpose, neurolytic medications are deposited or radiofrequency denervation performed.

A successful lumbar sympathetic block is confirmed with a 2-3°C increase in the temperature of the affected limb.

Complications

Generic complications include: infection, bleeding/bruising, allergy/anaphylaxis, injection soreness/exacerbation of pain.

Trauma can occur due to the needle used: nerve injury (lumbar nerve roots), vascular injury (iliac vessels), pneumothorax, injury to retroperitoneal organs.

There are also risks due to the medications used:

- Generic — local anaesthetic toxicity, systemic and local effects of steroids.
- Medication deposited in the correct site, but still producing unwanted effects — e.g. retrograde/failed ejaculation, genitofemoral neuralgia, lumbar plexus block.
- Medication deposited in the wrong site — e.g. accidental intravascular injections, accidental epidural/intrathecal injections.

Key Points

- The lumbar sympathetic ganglia provide sympathetic innervation to the lower limbs.
- This can be blocked for pain and vascular indications.
- Blocks can be temporary or permanent.
- The procedure is conducted at the L2/L3 level.
- Risks can be generic, due to the needle, or due to the medications used.

References

1. Alexander CE, Dulebohn SC. Lumbar sympathetic block. StatPearls [Internet], 2017. StatPearls Publishing.

Chapter 30

Injection therapy for chronic pain — coeliac plexus block

Shyam Balasubramanian

Applied anatomy

The coeliac plexus is present at the level of the L1 vertebra and is located anterior to the aorta and posterior to the pancreas (remember the mnemonic A to A and P to P), in front of the crura of the diaphragm (■ Figure 30.1).

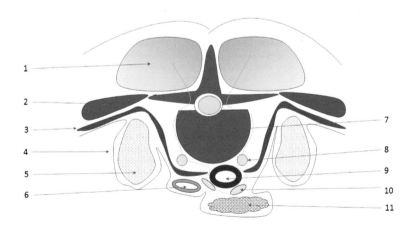

Figure 30.1. The coeliac plexus: 1. Erector spinae muscle; 2. Twelfth rib; 3. Diaphragm; 4. Peritoneum; 5. Kidney; 6. Inferior vena cava; 7. L1 vertebral body; 8. Sympathetic chain; 9. Aorta; 10. Coeliac plexus; 11. Pancreas.

The plexus comprises three pairs of ganglions:

- Coeliac ganglion.
- Superior mesenteric ganglion.
- Aorticorenal ganglion along with a meshwork of nerve fibres.

Sympathetic fibres from T5 to T12 and parasympathetic fibres from the vagus form the afferent fibres to the plexus. Efferent fibres from the plexus innervate all the non-pelvic abdominal viscera.

Indications

Chronic non-pelvic abdominal pain — a commonly described indication is abdominal pain secondary to pancreatic cancer. In view of the risks involved, generally a neurolytic technique is reserved for cancer pain management.

Contraindications

Relative contraindications include:

- Local infection.
- Altered coagulation, etc.

Technique

Preparation is key — the 4Ps:

- Preparation of the patient (pre-procedural assessment, consent).
- Preparation of the procedure room (monitoring, access to resuscitation facilities, medications, trained assistant).
- Preparation of the site (positioning, asepsis).
- Performance of the block.

Intravenous access and standard monitoring (ECG, blood pressure, pulse oximetry) should be in place.

A coeliac plexus block should be performed with fluoroscopy, a CT scanner, ultrasound and is endoscopy-guided. The approaches used are the anterior para-aortic approach and the posterior para-aortic approach.

The posterior para-aortic approach is usually performed under fluoroscopy guidance. With the patient in the prone position, under fluoroscopy guidance, the body of the L1 vertebra and twelfth ribs are identified. After skin infiltration with local anaesthetic at the inferior border of the twelfth rib, about 6-8cm from the midline, the spinal needle is introduced lateral to medial, aiming for the anterior aspect of the L1 vertebral body. Once the needle is in contact with the vertebral body, the fluoroscope is positioned to show the lateral view. The anteroposterior view is for the direction and the lateral view is for depth. The tip of the needle is advanced by another 1cm to pierce the prevertebral fascia. The fluoroscope is moved back to an anteroposterior view. Contrast is injected to demonstrate smooth cephalo-cranial spread, anterior to the aorta. Commonly, bilateral blocks are performed. A transaortic approach, where the needle goes through the aorta to its anterior surface, has also been described.

The anterior para-aortic approach is used in patients who cannot lay prone, usually due to advanced disease. The procedure is performed with fluoroscopy, a CT scanner and ultrasound guidance. The T12/L1 vertebral body is identified, and similar to the posterior technique, the needle is navigated until the tip reaches anterior to the aorta/diaphragm. Invariably, the needle may penetrate viscera including stomach, intestines and liver. Patients with terminal illness will tolerate the procedure better, but there is a higher risk due to the damage to abdominal organs.

If the coeliac plexus block is for diagnostic purpose or for benign conditions, local anaesthesia +/- steroids are deposited after careful negative aspiration. If the block is for a therapeutic purpose, neurolytic medication such as alcohol is deposited.

Complications

Generic complications include: infection, bleeding/bruising, allergy/anaphylaxis, injection soreness/exacerbation of pain.

Trauma can occur due to the needle used: nerve injury (lumbar nerve roots), vascular injury (aorta, inferior vena cava), pneumothorax, injury to retroperitoneal organs.

There are also risks due to the medications used:

- Generic — local anaesthetic toxicity, systemic and local effects of steroids.
- Medication deposited in the correct site, but still producing unwanted effects — e.g. orthostatic hypotension, diarrhoea.
- Medication deposited in the wrong site — e.g. accidental intravascular injections, accidental epidural/intrathecal injections.

Key Points

- The coeliac plexus innervates the non-pelvic abdominal viscera.
- The plexus is located anterior to the aorta and posterior to the pancreas.
- It is mainly blocked for cancer pain management.
- The procedure is conducted at the L1 level.
- Risks can be generic, due to the needle, or due to the medications used.

References

1.   John RS, Dixon B, Shienbaum R. Celiac plexus block. StatPearls [Internet], 2020. StatPearls Publishing. https://www.ncbi.nlm.nih.gov/books/NBK531469/. Accessed on 8th July 2020.

Chapter 31

Infusion therapies in chronic pain management

Shyam Balasubramanian

When a pain condition is not responding to oral medications or is not amenable to be managed with targeted procedures, intravenous infusions of different pharmacological agents have been tried for pain relief. Various non-opioid intravenous infusions have been tried with mixed results. Medications used in the infusion include lidocaine, magnesium, ketamine, bisphosphonates and phentolamine. Some infusions such as lidocaine and magnesium have been studied widely while others have limited evidence to support their routine use.

Indications

Indications include: chronic widespread pain, neuropathic pain, complex regional pain syndrome, headache and orofacial pain.

Lidocaine

Mechanism

Voltage-gated sodium channels have been implicated in the pathogenesis and maintenance of neuropathic and inflammatory pain conditions. In these pain conditions, proliferation of the sodium channels can cause random firing of pain signals from the site of injury, dorsal root ganglion and even from the uninjured neurons. Lidocaine acts by blocking the sodium channels in the neuronal cell membrane.

Dose

The dose is 3-5mg/kg over 30-60 minutes.

Side effects

Side effects include: blood pressure changes, arrhythmias, nausea and vomiting, numbness and tingling, dizziness, headache and seizures.

Magnesium

Mechanism

Excitatory amino acid glutamate is involved in the pain pathway. In chronic pain, activation of the NMDA glutamate receptors increases sustained neuronal depolarisation. NMDA receptors increase the excitatory transmission along the pain pathway in the dorsal horn of the spinal cord (wind-up phenomenon) and alters the cellular signalling pathways that accentuate the responsiveness of nociceptive neurons (central sensitization phenomenon). Magnesium is an NMDA antagonist. It is a physiological blocker of NMDA calcium channels, blocking calcium influx into the cell and contributing to secondary neuronal changes.

Dose

The dose is 30-50mg/kg over 60 minutes.

Side effects

Side effects include: flushing, nausea, sedation, depressed cardiac conduction, hypotension and muscle weakness.

Ketamine

Mechanism

Excitatory amino acid glutamate is involved in the pain pathway. In chronic pain, activation of the NMDA glutamate receptors increases sustained neuronal depolarisation. NMDA receptors increase the excitatory transmission along the pain pathway in the dorsal horn of the spinal cord (wind-up phenomenon) and alters the cellular signalling pathways that accentuate the responsiveness of nociceptive neurons (central sensitization phenomenon). Ketamine is an antagonist at NMDA receptors.

Dose

The dose is 0.3-0.5mg/kg over 30-60 minutes.

Side effects

Side effects include: hallucinations and tachyarrhythmias.

Key Points

- Various chemicals have been used as intravenous infusions for resistant widespread pain.
- Lidocaine infusions are commonly used in fibromyalgia; they block the voltage-gated sodium channels.
- It is vital to use these infusions as part of multimodal management with significant education on self-management strategies. Quality of life improvement outcome measures should be used and audited during the use of these infusions.

References

1.   Kosharskyy B, Almonte W, Shaparin N, *et al.* Intravenous infusions in chronic pain management. *Pain Physician* 2013; 16: 231-49.

2.   Kim YH, Lee PB, Oh TK. Is magnesium sulfate effective for pain in chronic postherpetic neuralgia patients comparing with ketamine infusion therapy? *J Clin Anesth* 2015; 27(4): 296-300.

Chapter 32

Ultrasound in chronic pain

Shyam Balasubramanian

Ultrasound has a role in diagnostic and therapeutic interventional procedures in pain management. Injection techniques based on landmarks are unreliable and can be difficult in subjects with an altered body habitus. Fluoroscopic guidance improves precision but deposition of injectate in the correct soft tissue plane may not always be possible. Ultrasound enables visualisation of soft tissues including nerves and blood vessels. It is portable, cost-effective and avoids the risk of radiation.

The physics of ultrasound

Ultrasound is high-pitched sound at a frequency above that of human hearing, ranging between 2MHz and 15MHz. The fundamental concept of ultrasound technology is 'echo formation'. The basic elements to form a sonographic image are a source for ultrasound, a reflector, a receiver and technology to convert the echo signals to an image. The transducer sends the signals (source) as well as collects the reflected signals (receiver). The human body forms the reflector. Depending on the composition of tissues, different sonographic patterns are produced.

A common mode used in interventional pain medicine is the 'B-mode', where B refers to brightness. Colour Doppler imaging is useful to identify blood vessels.

Ultrasound transducers

In interventional pain medicine, linear and curvilinear arrays are commonly used. Linear types provide undistorted images whereas curvilinear types scan a wider area with some image distortion. High-frequency linear transducers (10-15MHz) have a lower penetration, but a higher resolution and are ideal for superficial structures such as peripheral nerve blocks. Low-frequency curvilinear transducers (2-5MHz) have a better penetration, but a lower resolution and are ideal for deeper structures such as the spine.

When the transducer is placed across the anatomical structure it is a short axis view or transverse view. If it is placed along the direction of the anatomical structure it is a long axis view or longitudinal view.

In relation to the transducer, the needle can be introduced in two approaches, in-plane and out-of-plane.

Sonographic appearances

Tissues of different acoustic impedances when they lie adjacent to one another form a 'tissue interface'. The ultrasound beam passing through the tissue interface is variably reflected, refracted and scattered, resulting in different sonographic patterns:

* Anechoic — fluids, fat and bone appear dark.
* Hypoechoeic — muscles appear grey with striations.
* Hyperechoeic — fascial planes, bone surfaces, dense ligaments, etc. create a 'whitish' reflection. Neural structures appear differently depending on their location and the arrangement of fascicles. At the nerve root level, nerves are predominantly anechoic (e.g. interscalene brachial plexus); peripheral nerves have a honeycomb appearance (e.g. femoral nerve).

Highly reflective surfaces such as bone reflect almost the entire ultrasound beam resulting in the area behind this interface appearing dark, and this is described as an 'acoustic shadow'. Between the bones, the ultrasound beam passes through soft tissues producing different sonographic patterns, described as an 'acoustic window'. For example, ribs produce an acoustic shadow and the intercostal muscles, pleura and lung shadows appear in the acoustic window.

Limitations

A thorough understanding of the relevant anatomy is mandatory to safely perform ultrasound-guided interventions. Suboptimal resolution of images of deeper anatomical structures, and difficulties in visualising beyond bony structures limit its application. Whilst it is relatively easy to visualise the spread of injectate in superficial injections, an inability to use radiographic contrasts may make it difficult to rule out intravascular spread, particularly in deeper injection procedures such as lumbar nerve root blocks.

Key Points

- Ultrasound helps to visualise soft tissues; it is portable and avoids the risk of radiation.
- Ultrasound at a frequency between 2 and 15MHz is commonly used.
- High-frequency linear transducers give a better resolution but a limited penetration.
- Low-frequency curvilinear transducers give a better penetration but a limited resolution.
- Limitations include a difficulty in visualising the needle in deeper structures and beyond bone.

References

1. Balasubramanian S, Rayen AA. The use of ultrasound in pain management. In: *Ultrasound in anesthesia, critical care and pain management*. Arthurs G, Nicholls B, Eds. Cambridge University Press, 2017: 332.

2. Bandikatla VB, Narayanan S, Balasubramanian S. Introduction to ultrasound-guided blocks. In: *Interventional pain management: a practical approach*. Jaypee Brothers Medical Publishers, 2016: 431.

Chapter 33

Radiation — physics and risks

Arul James and Thanthullu Vasu

Radiation is widely used in the diagnosis and treatment of various medical conditions. Anaesthetists are exposed to ionising radiation while anaesthetising for interventional radiology procedures; pain physicians are exposed to ionising radiation during X-ray-guided interventions for chronic pain.

Radiation is the process of emission or propagation of energy through space or matter. The different types of radiation include light, heat, sound, microwaves, particle and electromagnetic radiation.

Why is ionising radiation harmful?

Ionising radiation has sufficient energy to remove one or more electrons from an atom, which makes the atom ionised. It includes high-frequency electromagnetic radiation such as X-rays, gamma rays and particle radiation (alpha particles, beta particles, neutrons, positrons). It can be natural or artificial.

Ionising radiation is harmful to living cells because it causes cell death both directly, by breaking cellular chemical bonds including DNA, and indirectly, by the formation of free radicals secondary to ionisation of water molecules which are present in the body.

Measurements in radiation

Radiation energy is measured in electronvolt (eV). One eV is the energy carried by one particle of radiation, which is 1.6×10^{-19} joules. Radiation energy of visible light is around 2eV, diagnostic X-ray is around 100keV and radiotherapy ranges around 20MeV.

Linear energy transfer (LET) is the amount of energy transferred per unit distance by the ionising radiation to the material traversed. It is measured in kiloelectronvolt per micrometre (keV/µm). X-rays and gamma rays have a low LET, while alpha and beta particles have a high LET.

Absorbed dose (D_T) is used to quantify the radiation energy absorbed by a unit mass of human tissue. The unit for absorbed dose is Gray (Gy), where one Gray is equivalent to one Joule of energy absorbed by one kilogram of tissue. However, different types of ionising radiation produce different biological effects; an equivalent dose (H_T) is used to quantify this relative different deterministic biological effect by using a radiation-specific weighting factor (W_R) in addition to the dose absorbed by tissue (D_T):

$$H_T = D_T \times W_R$$

The unit for equivalent dose is Sievert (Sv). In contrast to an equivalent dose which measures the deterministic effect, the effective dose is a measure of the stochastic effect of ionising radiation on the whole body, which is used for assessing radiological protection. The unit for effective dose is also Sievert.

Risks of ionising radiation

Medical use of ionising radiation has potential risks for patients, physicians and operating department personnel. Hence, we should have an adequate understanding of the basic physics of radiation, the risks involved and how to avoid them. The latest safety guidelines to be followed during medical exposure of patients to ionising radiation are the Ionising Radiation (Medical Exposure) Regulations 2017 (Amended 2018) (IRMER). The Regulations state that each exposure should be justified and we must ensure that the benefits outweigh the risks; unintended medical exposure should be kept to the minimum and the radiation dose kept as low as reasonably practicable.

Stochastic effects of ionising radiation

Exposure to ionising radiation can produce stochastic and deterministic effects. Stochastic effects are those that occur by chance and include the development of cancer and hereditary effects. There is no threshold for developing these effects and the risk increases proportionally with increasing dose of radiation. Some tissues like lungs, the gastrointestinal tract and bone marrow are more prone to carcinogenesis. It has been estimated that diagnostic medical radiation causes around 700 excess cancer deaths per year and 0.6% of all cancers are caused by diagnostic radiation in the UK. The typical radiation doses and the risk of cancer from common radiological diagnostic procedures are outlined in ■ Table 33.1 below.

Table 33.1. Typical radiation doses and the risk of cancer from common radiological diagnostic procedures.

Diagnostic procedure	Typical effective doses (mSv)	Equivalent period of natural background radiation*	Lifetime additional risk of fatal cancer per examination**
Chest (single PA film)	0.02	3 days	1 in a million
Skull	0.07	11 days	1 in 300,000
Abdomen	0.7	4 months	1 in 30,000
Lumbar spine	1.3	7 months	1 in 15,000
CT head	2	1 year	1 in 10,000
CT chest	8	3.6 years	1 in 2500
CT abdomen/pelvis	10	4.5 years	1 in 2000

* UK average = 2.2mSv per year: regional averages range from 1.5-7.5mSv per year.
** Approximate lifetime risk for patients 16 to 69 years old. For paediatric patients, multiply risks by about 2; for geriatric patients, divide risks by about 5.

Deterministic effects of ionising radiation

Deterministic effects have a threshold dose, below which there are no effects. Above this threshold dose, the severity of deterministic effects increases as the dose increases. Actively dividing cells like gastrointestinal mucous membranes, bone marrow, or gonads are more radio-sensitive. In contrast, nerves and muscles are radio-resistant. In-utero exposure can result in foetal death, childhood cancer and mental retardation.

Acute radiation syndrome

Acute radiation syndrome (ARS) is caused by irradiation to the entire body by a high dose of penetrating radiation in a very short period of time (■ Table 33.2). Mild symptoms may occur at doses of 0.3-0.7 Gray.

Table 33.2. Acute radiation syndrome.

Syndrome	Dose	Clinical features	Recovery
Hematopoietic	>0.7Gy	• Anorexia, nausea, vomiting, fever, malaise. • Fall in cell counts.	• In most cases, bone marrow cells will begin to repopulate the marrow.
Gastrointestinal	>10Gy	• Anorexia, nausea, vomiting, diarrhoea. • Fever, dehydration, electrolyte imbalance.	• Death occurs within 2 weeks of exposure.
Cardiovascular/ central nervous system	>50Gy	• Nervousness, confusion. • Convulsions, coma.	• Death occurs within 3 days of exposure.

Key Points

- Ionising radiation is harmful and causes cell death; directly by breaking chemical bonds including DNA and indirectly by forming free radicals from water.
- One eV is the energy carried by one particle of radiation, equalling 1.6 x 10^{-19} joules.
- Linear energy transfer (LET) is the energy transferred per unit distance (keV/μm). X-rays and gamma rays have a low LET while alpha and beta particles have a high LET.
- An equivalent dose is $H_T = D_T \times W_R$, measured in Sievert.
- Ionising radiation has stochastic and deterministic effects.
- Acute radiation syndrome (ARS) is due to a high dose of penetrating radiation to the entire body in a very short period of time.

References

1. Berrington de González A, Darby S. Risk of cancer from diagnostic X-rays: estimates for the UK and 14 other countries. *Lancet* 2004; 363(9406): 345-51.

2. Parkin D, Darby S. Cancers in 2010 attributable to ionising radiation exposure in the UK. *Br J Cancer* 2011; 105: S57-65.

3. Ionising Radiation (Medical Exposure) Regulations 2017: guidance. Guidance on the Ionising Radiation (Medical Exposure) Regulations 2017 for employers and health professionals who carry out medical radiological procedures. Department of Health and Social Care, 2018. https://www.gov.uk/government /publications/ionising-radiation-medical-exposure-regulations-2017-guidance. Accessed on 10th July 2020.

4. Patient dose information: guidance. Public Health England, 2008. https://www.gov.uk/government/ publications/medical-radiation-patient-doses/patient-dose-information-guidance. Accessed on 10th July 2020.

5. A brochure for physicians; Acute radiation syndrome. https://www.cdc.gov/nceh/radiation/ emergencies/pdf/ars.pdf. Accessed on 16th September 2020.

Chapter 34

Complementary therapies

Thanthullu Vasu

Complementary therapies are not part of conventional medical care but are used alongside to aid the multimodal and comprehensive pain management plan. All these therapies should include education of chronic pain management strategies in a holistic manner. Complementary therapy is used alongside conventional medical treatments, whereas alternative medicine is used instead of conventional treatments.

A few of the more common techniques that are used as complementary therapy in the pain management plan include: acupuncture, TENS machines, breathing techniques, yoga, tai chi, aromatherapy, art therapy, hypnosis, etc. Some form of cognitive behavioural therapy, mindfulness and/or acceptance commitment therapy is always included. There is much to be gained from the expertise of these skilled healthcare practitioners.

The main challenges to this approach include:

- To realise their limitations and understand that it is a part of the multimodal management.
- To find the right healthcare practitioner who can do it as part of the biopsychosocial model and has an expertise in chronic pain management.

Acupuncture

Various theories have been proposed regarding the mechanisms of acupuncture in chronic pain: stimulation and neuromodulation of the

175

nervous system; release of endorphins; activation of the descending inhibitory pathways; reducing activation of the pain matrix in the brain. It is commonly used in neck pain, headaches, back pain, fibromyalgia and other pain conditions. The authors have noticed that acupuncture helps in creating a rapport and engaging challenging patients in the biopsychosocial model and reducing medication intake.

In a randomised study on the use of acupuncture in headaches, it was noted that the acupuncture group made 25% fewer doctor visits, used 15% less medicines and had 15% less sick days.

The low back pain guidelines from NICE do NOT recommend acupuncture in low back pain.

The NICE headache guidelines recommend a course of up to ten sessions of acupuncture over 5-8 weeks for the prophylactic treatment of chronic tension-type headaches.

TENS machines

Transcutaneous electrical nerve stimulators (TENS) are used in most NHS pain services as part of the pain management strategy and are a popular treatment modality. The mechanism of action is attributed to the gate control theory of pain. Although we have found them to be of benefit, the NICE guidelines do NOT recommend a TENS machine for low back pain.

A previous Cochrane review analysed 124 studies and concluded that the analgesic effectiveness of TENS machines still remains uncertain. This was proposedly due to an inadequate methodology and reporting in these studies.

Relaxation, distraction and breathing strategies

Relaxation and distraction strategies can be very useful in chronic pain management. Guided imagery and breathing techniques are commonly used and are recommended by NICE guidelines for widespread pain. Breathing techniques can be taught face-to-face or can be recommended by apps such as Breathe2relax. Deep diaphragmatic breathing is a commonly used technique and is proposed to reduce sympathomimetic amines during a flare-up if practised well before. Paediatric chronic pain clinics rely heavily on breathing strategies as part of the multimodal management.

Yoga and tai-chi

There are individual studies but a proper evidence base and meta-analyses are lacking at the present time.

Hypnosis

Hypnosis has been tried by many but the evidence base is limited at the present time.

Art therapies

Various forms of art are used in pain services but these need to be evaluated. These include: painting, knitting, expressive writing, etc. Most of these treatments have a NNH (number needed to harm) of zero and are worth including as a multimodal package of treatment, provided the message on self-management is well instilled in these sessions.

Massage

Massage is proposed to be of help by direct muscle relaxation, enhancement of parasympathetic activity, activation of the inhibitory pathway and indirectly through the reduction of stress. Unfortunately, there is a restricted evidence base at the present time and patients must be advised carefully to make sure they are referred to qualified practitioners. Massage should be used to enhance self-management strategies rather than letting passive dependence develop.

Key Points

- Complementary therapies are used *alongside* conventional treatments; alternative therapies are used *instead* of conventional treatments.
- Acupuncture is not recommended for low back pain (NICE guidelines), but is recommended for chronic tension-type headaches.
- NICE does not recommend a TENS machine for low back pain.

References

1. Hart J. Complementary therapies for chronic pain management. *J Altern Complem Therapies* 2008; 4: 64-8.

2. Vickers AJ, Rees RW, Zollman CE, *et al.* Acupuncture of chronic headache disorders in primary care: randomised controlled trial and economic analysis. *Health Technol Assess* 2004; 8(48): iii, 1-35.

3. Low back pain and sciatica in over 16s: assessment and management. NICE clinical guideline, NG59. London: National Institute for Health and Care Excellence, 2016. https://www.nice.org.uk/guidance/ng59. Accessed on 6th July 2020.

4. Headaches in over 12s: diagnosis and management. NICE clinical guideline, CG150. London: National Institute for Health and Care Excellence, 2012. https://www.nice.org.uk/guidance/cg150. Accessed on 6th July 2020.

5. Nnoaham KE, Kumbang J. Transcutaneous electrical nerve stimulation (TENS) for chronic pain. *Cochrane Database Syst Rev* 2014; Issue 7: CD003222.

6. Chronic fatigue syndrome/myalgic encephalomyelitis (or encephalopathy): diagnosis and management. NICE clinical guideline, CG53. London: National Institute for Health and Care Excellence, 2007. https://www.nice.org.uk/guidance/cg53. Accessed on 6th July 2020.

Chapter 35

Physiotherapy in chronic pain

Thanthullu Vasu

Physiotherapists work with chronic pain sufferers to identify and maximise their ability to move and function. They form an important part of the chronic pain multidisciplinary team. They achieve a better quality of life through self-management strategies and increasing levels of activity by pacing strategies. They are an integral part of pain management programmes to help in a patient's rehabilitation and functional restoration.

The Core Standards for Pain Management Services in the UK recommends that any pain service should include a Health and Care Professionals Council (HCPC) registered physiotherapist. It also suggests that they should be additionally trained in cognitive behavioural therapy (CBT) principles of pain management.

Most senior physiotherapists also have an expertise in acceptance and commitment therapy (ACT), graded exposure and goal setting, listening and advanced communication skills, and motivational interviewing.

Physiotherapists have a huge expertise in the triaging and assessment of chronic pain. Most triage services in the UK include an extended scope physiotherapist. They use the biopsychosocial principles in triage to allocate patients to the best possible resource available in the pain service.

Physiotherapists are vital in a chronic pain service to offer:

- Education — patient education to allay fears of chronic pain is important to gain a good rapport and engage them in a comprehensive self-management pathway.

- Exercises — paced and gradual exercises are the key to recovery. It is important to convey the message that "hurt does not mean harm". Ruling out diagnostic causes and educating patients before exercise intervention should be done to gain their compliance in continuing the exercises.
- Changing behavioural patterns — it is important to look at patient behaviour and their response to chronic pain; adapting to physical sensations and achieving healthy levels of activity is the goal to recovery.
- An important role in any pain management programme. They may also run specific groups such as back pain classes.
- Complementary therapies such as a TENS machine, acupuncture, etc. Some are trained to be independent prescribers. Pain management programmes often include yoga, tai chi, gym classes, mindfulness-based breathing exercises — all of which can be delivered by physiotherapists.
- Manual therapies such as soft tissue release, massage, etc., as part of a multimodal package, but always with a view to educating the patient regarding self-management and activity.

Physiotherapists may also use desensitization strategies in chronic neuropathic pain. In paediatric chronic pain clinics, they are vital in inculcating the distraction and relaxation strategies for pain management.

Key Points

- Physiotherapy maximises the ability to move and function.
- They are an integral part of pain service and pain management programmes.
- NICE guidelines recommend physiotherapy and exercises for many chronic pain conditions including low back pain.
- Physiotherapists have excellent skills in triage services and in the assessment of chronic pain.

References

1. Core Standards for Pain Management Services in the UK. Faculty of Pain Medicine of the Royal College of Anaesthetists. https://fpm.ac.uk/standards-publications-workforce/core-standards. Accessed on 10th July 2020.

Chapter 36

Psychology in chronic pain

Thanthullu Vasu

Comprehensive multidisciplinary pain management services always include psychology and value its role in self-management strategies. A low mood is common in chronic pain. Various studies have shown that depression is the third most common reason for consultation with a general practitioner and is the most common mood complaint. Depression and chronic pain are closely linked but their association is usually underestimated. It is said that around 40-60% of chronic pain patients suffer with depression. The outcomes are much poorer if they coexist rather than treating alone.

Pain can be a common symptom of an anxiety disorder. Chronic pain can itself cause anxiety regarding the health condition, its diagnosis and prognosis, and with regards to the treatment modalities.

'Pain catastrophisation' is a commonly used term in pain clinics; 'catastrophisation' is an exaggerated fear of pain or pain experience. It is associated with a lack of confidence and control, and leads to poor outcomes. Education and explanation play a major role in the outcome in these patients. Good communication skills also play a great role in helping these patients to understand the need to avoid irrational fears with regards to chronic pain.

The fear-avoidance theory is popularly used in pain services to explain why fear can cause limited mobility and disengagement with activity and lead to disuse. Normally, after injury, we manage our fear and confront and recover; whereas in susceptible patients, the pain experience and fear can lead to a vicious cycle and cause persistent pain.

Sleep interruption and poor sleep hygiene plays a major role in the persistence of chronic pain. Education regarding sleep hygiene is a vital component of the chronic pain management plan. Furthermore, medications for pain can cause poor-quality sleep.

Yellow flags

Yellow flags are psychosocial factors that are indicative for long-term chronicity and disability. These include: a negative attitude that pain is harmful and disabling, fear avoidance and reduced activity, an expectation of passive treatments, a tendency for depression and social withdrawal, and social/financial problems.

Assessing and measuring mood

The Hospital Anxiety and Depression Scale (HADS) has been commonly used in many pain services to score anxiety and depression levels. It is easy to score and asks patients to score how they felt in the previous week. A score of 8-10 is considered borderline; a score of more than 11 will need to be monitored and treated appropriately.

Various other scores have been used to assess the psychological status of a patient. Each pain service uses their own preferred sets of scores to look at the diagnosis, treatment pathway and management. It helps to assess outcomes in terms of quality of life improvement of patients. Other scores include:

- Brief Pain Inventory (BPI).
- EuroQol score for quality assessment in various dimensions (EQ-5D).
- Pain Anxiety Symptoms Scale (PASS).
- Survey of Pain Attitudes (SOPA).
- Chronic Pain Coping Inventory (CPCI).
- Chronic Pain Acceptance Questionnaire CPAQ).
- Pain Catastrophising Scale (PCS), etc.

Talking therapies

All pain services offer some form of talking therapy; in the community, self-referral schemes might also be available. Some forms of talking therapy may include:

- Cognitive behavioural therapy (CBT).
- Improving Access to Psychological Therapies (IAPT) — NHS initiative to improve mental health.
- Psychodynamic therapy.
- Group therapy.
- Counselling.

Cognitive behavioural therapy (CBT)

CBT is based on the fact that our thoughts, feelings and behaviour are interconnected. The goal is to change the way patients think (cognitive) and/or what they do (behavioural) so that they change the way they feel.

CBT aims to identify challenging unhelpful thoughts; through graded exposure, it can reduce unhelpful behaviours and remove unnecessary fears.

Mindfulness therapy

Acting with awareness is the goal in mindfulness; this leads to positive thinking rather than catastrophising. It helps the patient to be fully present and be aware of where they are and what they are doing and to not be overwhelmed by what happens outside. A meditative approach can help in distraction and relaxation strategies. Awareness is created in all senses which can affect the present state of mind through thoughts and emotions.

Mindfulness-based stress reduction and mindfulness-based cognitive therapy are incorporated in many pain management services.

Acceptance and commitment therapy (ACT)

ACT encourages embracing our thoughts and feelings, leading to commitment and behaviour change strategies. Rather than controlling thoughts and feelings as in CBT, ACT teaches us how to notice, accept and embrace them.

ACT might not necessarily aid a patient to accept pain but it will help in accepting unwanted experiences due to pain.

The six core principles of ACT that help to develop psychological flexibility include:

- Cognitive defusion.
- Acceptance.
- Being in the present moment.
- Self as context.
- Discovering values.
- Committed action.

Paediatric chronic pain clinics largely use metaphors as a way of explaining the basis of ACT in their consultations.

Psychological interventions should be used if there is a possibility of changing the outcome and improving the quality of life for a patient. It is very clear that pain behaviours and coping styles determine functioning and quality of life, more significantly than the pain intensity. It is therefore vital to include multidisciplinary input at the early possible opportunity for chronic pain patients.

Key Points

- Depression and anxiety are common in chronic pain patients.
- Catastrophisation is an exaggerated fear of pain.
- Fear avoidance worsens the disability in chronic pain.
- Yellow flags — psychosocial factors that are indicative of chronicity and disability.
- CBT — thoughts, feelings and behaviours are interconnected.
- Mindfulness — being aware of the present only.
- ACT — cognitive defusion, acceptance, being present, self, values and commitment.

References

1. Surah A, Baranidharan G, Morley S. Chronic pain and depression. *Contin Educ Anaesth Critical Care Pain* 2014; 14(2): 85-9.

2. Vlaeyen JW, Linton SJ. Fear-avoidance and its consequences in chronic musculoskeletal pain: a state of the art. *Pain* 2000; 85(3): 317-32.

3. Samanta J, Kendall J, Samanta A. Chronic low back pain. *BMJ* 2003; 326(7388): 535.

4. NHS conditions: Cognitive behavioural therapy. www.nhs.uk/conditions/cognitive-behavioural-therapy-cbt/. Accessed on 10th July 2020.

5. Gauntlett-Gilbert J, Brook P. Living well with chronic pain: the role of pain-management programmes. *BJA Educ* 2018; 18(1): 3-7.

Chapter 37

Pain management programmes

Pradeep Mukund Ingle

Pain management programmes (PMPs) are an important part of pain services; they are based on cognitive behavioural principles and involve a group programme with multiple healthcare professionals. They promote physical, social and emotional wellbeing, and a behaviour change in order to improve the quality of life (QOL) in patients with persistent pain.

The aims of a PMP

A PMP aims to provide skills and resources to patients for their self-management (ability to cope) of pain and to achieve as normal life as possible in patients with persistent pain by:

- Decreasing the emotional distress component in chronic pain.
- Reducing disability (physical) associated with chronic pain.
- Improving self-management.
- Decreasing their dependence on healthcare resources.

Structure

A PMP involves multiple healthcare professionals including pain physicians, physiotherapists, occupational therapists, specialist pain nurses and psychologists with a mixture of shared and some unique competencies amongst themselves. Other specialties such as pharmacists and previous participant patients as guides can also be involved to enhance the impact of a PMP.

There are four important aspects of a PMP:

- Education — on general health and wellbeing, pain physiology and psychology with an important focus on the self-management of pain.
- Guided physical therapy — management of activity with an exercise component that involves appropriate and realistic goal setting.
- Guided behavioural change — identifying unhelpful beliefs, thinking and habits to change a patient's behaviour with the intention of controlling the disability.
- Integration of learned skills in daily life — integrate the above in a practical way in daily life.

A PMP is usually delivered in a group format with 8-12 participants. A lack of skilled staff, resources and time reduces the overall effectiveness of a PMP. Usually the more time involved and the more intense the PMP is, the more chances there are of improving success rates.

A standard PMP

The British Pain Society (BPS) recommends approximately 12 half-day sessions (36 hours approximately); in clinical practice, usually this is spread over a 6 to 10-week period with 1 day a week of participation.

Variations in a PMP

An intensive residential PMP (15 to 20 days) can be delivered for patients who are significantly disabled or distressed. A specialist PMP needs some operational flexibility to inculcate individual psychology- and physiotherapy-based interventions, either before, during or after a PMP is completed to optimise the results. This is particularly important for patients with certain conditions such as chronic pelvic pain, facial pain or for young adults with chronic pain. A targeted early PMP is predominantly composed of physiotherapy- and psychology-based interventions that can be employed as a cost-effective strategy in the early stages.

Evidence

There is level 1 evidence of a PMP's effectiveness in people with persistent pain. In terms of improving the pain experience, mood, coping, activity levels, a negative outlook in chronic pain, cognitive PMPs offer a better efficacy in comparison with standard treatment or no treatment (level 1 evidence).

There is also some evidence that PMPs reduce the chances of patients presenting to the accident and emergency department or primary care with pain-related problems.

The incidence of patients being re-referred to specialist pain services and further use of pain medications are reduced with a PMP.

Outcomes

Outcomes from a PMP need to be evaluated. An improved quality of life and return to work are considered important goals.

Challenges

There is currently a restriction of services to access a PMP. For a PMP to be successful there are many practicalities to consider including the development of a multidisciplinary team and the system to maintain it.

Communication between primary care, referrers and the commissioning bodies can be challenging.

PMPs for children and adolescents are significantly scarce and in need of development.

Online and web-based technologies have been used in PMP delivery but these need to be evaluated for their evidence base in the near future.

Key Points

- A pain management programme (PMP) involves a multidisciplinary team with the aim of reducing a patient's distress and disability.
- A PMP is conducted as group therapy and has a high level of evidence.
- PMPs are recommended by NICE and the British Pain Society for a variety of chronic pain conditions.
- Challenges due to multidisciplinary staff availability and fiscal resources are overcome usually by enthusiastic staff with a passion to help chronic pain sufferers.

References

1. Guidelines for pain management programmes for adults. An evidence-based review prepared on behalf of the British Pain Society. The British Pain Society, 2013. https://www.britishpainsociety.org/static/uploads/resources/files/pmp2013_main_FINAL_v6.pdf. Accessed on 10th July 2020.
2. Wilkinson P, Whiteman R. Pain management programmes. *BJA Educ* 2017; 17(1): 10-5.

Chapter 38

Spinal cord stimulators and intrathecal pumps

Arul James and Thanthullu Vasu

Spinal cord stimulators (SCSs) for the management of chronic pain

A spinal cord stimulator is a mechanical device implanted into a patient's body to reduce chronic pain using small doses of electricity which are directly delivered to the nerves in the spinal column. It consists of electrodes, a pulse generator and connecting wires. The electrodes (leads) are placed in the dorsal epidural space and connected to the pulse generator by wires (cables). Some SCS systems may have an external device to change the programming of the SCS.

The history of SCSs

In 1965, Melzack and Wall described the gate control theory of pain. They proposed that non-painful stimulation of non-nociceptive neural pathways could inhibit the neural transmission of painful sensations to the brain. Shealy *et al* performed the first SCS in 1967 based on this principle. The initial SCSs were surgically placed under general anaesthesia and required a laminotomy or laminectomy. However, recent technology has enabled the minimally invasive percutaneous insertion of an SCS in an awake patient with local anaesthetic infiltration.

SCS multidisciplinary team

The insertion of an SCS should be delivered by a multidisciplinary team which includes pain physicians, psychologists, physiotherapists, nurse specialists in chronic pain, and spinal surgeons or neurosurgeons competent with using SCSs. The patient should undergo a thorough assessment because the selection criteria for the insertion of an SCS are important predictors of the long-term success of this treatment. The procedure is performed in an operating theatre environment. The pulse width, frequency and amplitude of the SCS can be adjusted to provide the most optimal pain relief possible.

Mechanism of action

It acts via neuromodulation using spinal and supra-spinal mechanisms. A small electrical field is created around the electrodes which are placed in the dorsal epidural space. The electric field stimulates the nerve fibres in the dorsal column of the spinal cord. This causes inhibition of wide dynamic range neurons, activation of inhibitory inter-neurons, activation of the descending inhibitory neuronal pathway and inhibition of efferent sympathetic output.

Indications for SCS

An SCS can be used in adults with the following chronic neuropathic pain conditions which have not responded to more conservative treatment: failed back surgery syndrome; complex regional pain syndrome (CRPS); pain associated with peripheral vascular disease; and refractory angina pectoris. The NICE recommendation is to consider this treatment modality when the pain score is persistently above 50mm in a 0-100mm visual analogue scale for more than 6 months despite conservative treatment of the above conditions.

Contraindications

There are absolute and relative contraindications for the insertion of a spinal cord stimulator. Absolute contraindications include infection at the site of insertion, sepsis or an uncontrolled bleeding disorder. Relative contraindications include the need for chronic anticoagulant therapy, and an immunosuppressive state.

Complications

The most common complication is lead migration. Device-related complications such as lead disconnection and problems with the battery are more common than biological complications such as infection, nerve injury, pain, epidural haematoma or fibrosis.

Intrathecal pumps: intrathecal drug delivery (ITDD) systems

Intrathecal pumps are surgically implanted mechanical devices which can deliver medicines into the intrathecal space. It consists of a pump and catheter. The pump contains the medicine and the catheter connects the pump to the subarachnoid space. The pump can be placed externally or it can be fully implanted in the body with a reservoir that can be refilled percutaneously. The pumps can deliver the medicine at a fixed rate or at a variable rate which can be programmed in the device.

Mechanism of action

Intrathecal pumps will deliver an adequate concentration of drugs in the dorsal horn of the spinal cord to produce effective analgesia. Hence, the dose required for effective analgesia is lower via intrathecal pumps compared with systemic administration of the same drug. The FDA approved drugs which can be delivered via ITDD systems include baclofen, morphine and ziconotide.

Indications

ITDD systems are indicated in the following chronic painful conditions which persist despite conservative management or for patients developing intolerable side effects from medications given via other routes of administration: cancer pain; chronic pancreatitis; failed back surgery syndrome; complex regional pain syndrome; and to relieve muscle spasms in cerebral palsy and multiple sclerosis.

Complications

Complications can be secondary to the surgical procedure, mechanical device or drugs used via the ITDD system. The surgical procedure can cause postoperative local infection, meningitis, bleeding and bruising. The mechanical device may stop working, may not be compatible with MRI, the catheter can get sheared, and may produce intrathecal granulomas, CSF leak and headache. Side effects due to the drugs used via the ITDD system include nausea, vomiting, dizziness, respiratory depression, muscular spasms, urinary retention and constipation.

Key Points

- SCS and ITDD systems are complex invasive interventions that need proper multidisciplinary evaluation and assessment.
- NICE guidance gives a high level of evidence for the use of SCS in refractory neuropathic pain.
- Opioids, baclofen and ziconotide are trialled via the ITDD systems.

References

1. Spinal cord stimulation for chronic pain of neuropathic or ischaemic origin. NICE technology appraisal guidance, TA159. London: National Institute for Health and Care Excellence, 2008. https://www.nice.org.uk/guidance/ta159/chapter/1-Guidance. Accessed on 6th July 2020.

2. Zhang TC, Janik JJ, Grill WM. Mechanisms and models of spinal cord stimulation for the treatment of neuropathic pain. *Brain Res* 2014; 1569: 19-31.

3. Eldabe A, Buchsher E, Duarte RV. Complications of spinal cord stimulation and peripheral nerve stimulation techniques: a review of the literature. *Pain* 2016; 17(2): 325-36.

4. Bottros MM, Christo PJ. Current perspectives on intrathecal drug delivery. *J Pain Res* 2014; 7: 615-26.

Chapter 39

Placebo and pain relief

Shyam Balasubramanian

Placebo is defined as any therapy or component of therapy used for its non-specific, psychological, or psycho-physiological effect, or that is used for its presumed specific effect, but is without specific activity for the condition being treated.

The placebo effect is the positive response that some patients/participants experience after receiving a placebo. The beneficial effect is either subjective

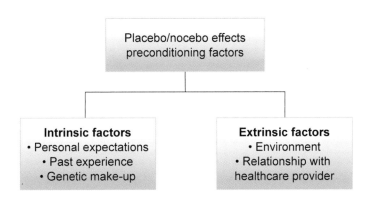

Figure 39.1. Preconditioning factors of placebo and nocebo effects.

or objective. The nocebo effect is the negative response that some patients/participants experience after receiving a placebo. Both the placebo and nocebo effects have certain preconditioning factors (■ Figure 39.1)

Mechanism of placebo analgesia

The placebo analgesic response is explained by:

- Psychological mechanisms (e.g. expectation of pain relief, conditioning).
- Neurobiological mechanisms (e.g. endorphins, dopamine, serotonin, cannabinoids).

The nocebo hyperalgesic response may be due to:

- Psychological mechanisms (e.g. anxiety and expectation of pain).
- Neurobiological mechanism (e.g. activation of the cholecystokininergic system).

The placebo/nocebo effects have been studied with functional magnetic resonance imaging (fMRI), which has revealed changes in the brain in areas such as the dorsolateral prefrontal cortex, the rostral anterior cingulate cortex and subcortical regions including the hypothalamus, amygdala and the periaqueductal gray.

The role of placebo

Placebo is used as follows:

- As controls in experimental studies to determine specific effects and to enable blinding.
- In placebo research to study the effects of placebo.
- As a tool in clinical practice. Ethical concerns continue to persist, and placebo is less likely to be promoted as a stand-alone intervention if there is an evidence-based alternative.

Key Points

- The placebo effect is a positive response to placebo.
- Nocebo is a negative response to placebo.
- Intrinsic patient factors and extrinsic environmental factors precondition these effects.
- The effects are explained by psychological and neurobiological mechanisms.

References

1. Balasubramanian S, Morley-Forster P, Bureau Y. Opioids and brain imaging: review. *J Opioid Manag* 2006; 2(3): 147-54.

2. Medoff ZM, Colloca L. Placebo analgesia: understanding the mechanisms. *Pain Manag* 2015; 5(2): 89-96.

Chapter 40

Pain management in drug abusers

Pradeep Mukund Ingle

Patients with a history of drug abuse pose a unique set of challenges with pain management. The drugs of abuse can either be prescription drugs or non-prescription drugs. Prescription drug abuse is commonly for drugs such as opioids, benzodiazepines, gabapentinoids, antidepressants and drugs for ADHD. Non-prescription drugs of abuse in the UK include alcohol, cannabis, ecstasy, ketamine, cocaine, heroin, etc.

Complex psychosocial issues, poor health, drug tolerance, physical dependence, addiction issues and some uncommon issues such as opioid-induced hyperalgesia are likely to complicate pain management in this group of the population. Besides this, they could also be on 'substitution therapy' drugs which are normally used to reduce the harm, craving and preoccupation associated with drugs of abuse.

Challenges in pain management in patients with drug abuse include:

* Associated anxiety and other psychological issues complicating optimal management.
* Increased pain sensitivity in acute and chronic settings needing more medical input.
* High rates of non-compliance with medical management.
* Self-discharge and self-medication are common.
* Associated drug issues such as dependence/tolerance for drugs of abuse, drug diversion and misuse.
* Pain management is often inadequate with an increased risk of relapse of addiction issues and recourse to the drugs of abuse.

- Unaccustomed healthcare staff with regards to the demands of this group of patients with a negative impact on the staff-patient relationship.
- Patients treated with 'substitution therapy' for their substance abuse with drugs such as methadone, buprenorphine (high dose) or oral naltrexone need specialist input for pain management which may not be easily available.
- All of the above issues require good communication with the patient and constant reassurance to gain their trust to comply with the overall management.

Pain management in acute pain settings

The following points need to be considered when managing patients with a drug abuse history:

- Prevention of withdrawal reactions from the drugs of abuse.
- Effective pain management for the ongoing pain condition with involvement of the acute pain team.
- Liaison with the multidisciplinary team (pain team, primary care doctor, pharmacist, substance abuse services, psychology services, etc.) as needed, to formulate a plan during hospitalisation and after discharge to address pain management as well as substance abuse issues.

Preventing withdrawal reactions:

- Prescription drugs especially opioids, gabapentinoids, etc., need to be continued during acute episodes of worsening pain that requires hospitalisation.
- If patients need PCA with opioids, consider background opioid infusions along with bolus PCA.
- Watch for withdrawal reactions to manage them optimally by involving multidisciplinary team members such as acute pain services, psychology and substance abuse support services.

Pain management:

- Multimodal management with opioid-sparing strategies can be beneficial. These include a combination of simple analgesics, local anaesthetic techniques, supplemental drugs such as magnesium, ketamine, clonidine and IV lignocaine infusions as per local protocols.
- Patient education, reassurance and empathic communication along with non-pharmacological interventions such as TENS and CBT.
- A plan should be documented for the management of pain as well as weaning of the pain medications that have a potential for dependence, addiction and abuse.
- Patients on methadone can divide it into 2-3 doses with additional doses titrated for analgesia.
- If a patient is on buprenorphine, a similar approach can be used as for methadone; alternatively, it can be discontinued and other opioids/alternatives can be used for analgesia.
- If the patient is on naltrexone (a long-acting opioid antagonist), it needs to be discontinued if opioids are likely to be needed for acute pain management, bearing in mind that there is heightened sensitivity for opioids in these patients for up to 6 days after stopping naltrexone. In pre-operative settings, it needs to be discontinued for 72 hours before surgery.

Pain management in chronic pain settings

There is evidence to suggest that people with substance abuse are more likely to consume opioids for their pain issues. However, this group of the population has complex physical and psychosocial issues. Hence, analgesics should only form a small part of wider self-management rather than the main focus of pain management.

Exercise, psychology-based interventions and rehabilitation should be prioritised for effective pain management. There is very little evidence to support the use of long-term opioids (especially for >120mg/day of oral morphine equivalent) for the management of chronic non-cancer pain and hence their use must be discouraged in view of their risks. Opioids may only be used as a short trial for a few weeks with a clear plan for discontinuation later.

Maintenance treatment for addiction can involve opioids such as methadone or buprenorphine which need titration and monitoring from specialist services. There should be a plan to de-escalate these opioids and gradually wean the patients off opioids in the long term.

Pain management in palliative care settings

Multimodal analgesia involving the titrated use of non-opioids, opioids and adjuvant medications is vital for effective pain management in palliative care.

Patients with a history of substance abuse should not be denied analgesia even if they require opioids for effective pain palliation. Specialist help and regular reviews are needed.

Opioids are likely to be needed in providing background analgesia as well as analgesia for breakthrough pain. Multimodal analgesia should be considered wherever possible.

Liaison between the palliative care team, psychology services and drug services should offer the necessary pain management along with preventing withdrawal reactions and providing psychological support.

Key Points

- Patients with a history of drug abuse can present with challenges in pain management in acute, chronic and palliative care settings.
- Preventing withdrawal reactions, along with multidisciplinary pain management forms a vital aspect of pain management in this group of patients.
- Emphatic communication, reassurance and patient education along with non-pharmacological management helps to improve patient outcomes.

References

1.   Substance misuse: acute pain management. Faculty of Pain Medicine of the Royal College of Anaesthetists. https://www.fpm.ac.uk/opioids-aware-opioids-addiction/substance-misuse-acute-pain-management. Accessed on 13th July 2020.

2.   Simpson GK, Jackson M. Perioperative management of opioid-tolerant patients. *BJA Educ* 2017; 17(4): 124-8.

3.   Substance misuse: chronic pain management. Faculty of Pain Medicine of the Royal College of Anaesthetists. https://fpm.ac.uk/opioids-aware-opioids-addiction/substance-misuse-chronic-pain-management. Accessed on 15th July 2020.

4.   Substance misuse: pain management in palliative care. Faculty of Pain Medicine of the Royal College of Anaesthetists. https://fpm.ac.uk/opioids-aware-opioids-addiction/substance-misuse-pain-management-palliative-care. Accessed on 15th July 2020.

Chapter 41

Pain management in intensive care

Ravindra Pochiraju and Mahesh Kodivalasa

Pain management in intensive care is complex; this is made further difficult by the challenges in communication and the physiological derangements affecting the metabolism of analgesic medications.

Severe or poorly managed pain induces a stress response and sympatho-adrenergic stimulation. This in turn leads to myocardial stress and a catabolic state in susceptible patients.

Systemic deleterious effects of pain include hyperglycaemia, immunosuppression, impaired wound healing, hypercoagulability and increased catabolism. All of these unwanted effects can lead to an increased length of intensive care, hospital stay and mortality.

Pharmacokinetic and pharmacodynamic problems in intensive care patients

In the ever-changing dynamic intensive care setting, multiple physiological derangements in critically ill patients deleteriously influence the pharmacology of drugs:

- Ileus — unpredictable absorption of orally administered drugs.
- Altered protein binding — increased free drug fractions (in hypoalbuminaemia).
- Deranged acid-base balance — affects the ionized and bound fraction of drugs.

- Altered splanchnic blood flow (shock states) — reduces phase 1 and 2 dependent metabolism.
- Organ dysfunction — hepatic and renal dysfunction reduces metabolism and excretion of drugs and their metabolites.
- Pharmacodynamic effects — alterations in the blood brain barrier result in an increased sensitivity to drug effects.

Common causes of pain in intensive care

- Constant background pain — surgical incisions, abdominal/chest drains, neuropathic pain (spinal cord injuries, Guillain-Barré syndrome, multiple sclerosis), fractures, soft tissue injuries, burns, pressure sores, etc.
- Intermittent/peri-procedural pain — central venous catheter placement, chest drain insertion, nasogastric tube insertion, position change, tracheal suctioning, physiotherapy, wound/burn dressing changes, etc.

Assessment of pain in intensive care

- Self-reporting of pain is the gold standard wherever possible.
- Commonly used pain assessment scales in patients who are able to communicate include the visual analogue scale, numerical rating scale and verbal rating scale.
- Commonly used pain scales for patients unable to communicate include the Behavioural Pain Scale and the Critical care Pain Observation Tool (CPOT), etc.
- The Behavioural Pain Scale cumulative score ranges from 3 to 12. A score of more than 6 requires adequate pain management.
- The Critical care Pain Observation Tool (CPOT) score ranges from 0 to 8. A score of more than 2 indicates pain that needs further evaluation and management.
- Age appropriate scales such as the FACES, COMFORT or FLACC scales should be used in children.

The principles of pain management in intensive care

- An analgesia first (A1) approach, emphasising analgesia before sedation should be practised.
- Effective management includes a holistic approach using a combination of pharmacological and non-pharmacological interventions. Non-pharmacological options include complementary/ alternative therapies such as music therapy, relaxation techniques, cold therapy, heat therapy, etc.
- A multimodal approach improves the quality of analgesia and reduces side effects.
- Medications and other approaches should be titrated to effect with regular reassessments and a patient-specific analgesic regimen.

Modalities of pain management in intensive care

- Systemic analgesia — opioids, paracetamol, NSAIDs, α2 agonists, gabapentinoids, ketamine, etc.
- Regional analgesia — epidural blocks, paravertebral blocks, peripheral nerve blocks, fascial pain blocks, wound catheters, etc.

Systemic analgesia:

- Systemic opioids are the mainstay of treatment for acute pain in critically ill patients. An initial bolus followed by a step-up approach of infusion is ideal for constant background pain relief. Significant adverse effects include ileus, hallucinations, hypotension, bradycardia and delirium.
- Paracetamol reduces opioid requirement and should be part of all multimodal regimens.
- NSAIDs have a limited use in intensive care patients due to the risks (renal dysfunction, bleeding) outweighing the benefits.
- Gabapentinoids are useful adjuncts in neuropathic pain (spinal cord injuries, Guillain-Barré syndrome, multiple sclerosis). Pregabalin has a better bioavailability when compared with gabapentin.

- α2 agonists (clonidine and dexmedetomidine) provide analgesia and sedation. They are also useful as adjuncts in alcohol/opioid-dependent patients.
- Ketamine (NMDA antagonist) provides analgesia and sedation, along with a useful opioid-sparing effect. It can be an effective third-line management option in difficult and challenging situations.

Regional analgesia:

- Offers excellent pain relief while avoiding opioid-induced side effects.
- The performance of regional analgesic techniques in intensive care is challenging owing to commonly associated factors such as sepsis, coagulopathy, sick and sedated patients.
- A high index of suspicion and close monitoring are necessary to detect any complications.
- There is an increased risk of regional analgesia catheter dislodgement due to repeated changes in position required for routine intensive care needs including mobilisation and physiotherapy.
- The pharmacodynamics and pharmacokinetics of local anaesthetics are altered due to the physiological and metabolic derangements seen in critically ill patients. This can lead to effects such as a delayed onset of action and local anaesthetic toxicity.

A selection of the indications for regional analgesia in intensive care include:

- Surgical — rib fractures (thoracic epidural, paraveterbral blocks, intercostal blocks); limb fractures/amputations (spinal/epidural, peripheral nerve blocks); thoracotomy (thoracic epidural/paravertebral blocks); laparotomy (TAP blocks, rectus sheath blocks, wound catheters).
- Non-surgical — acute pancreatitis (thoracic epidural, coeliac plexus blocks); ischaemic limb (sympathetic blocks).

Multimodal regimens incorporating appropriate systemic and regional analgesia offer optimum pain relief. Patients who are having major surgery such as a laparotomy can be managed with a combination of a titrated morphine infusion (in intubated patients), patient-controlled analgesia (PCA), paracetamol, TAP blocks (including subcostal blocks), rectus sheath blocks, and wound infusion catheters. Analgesic adjuncts such as clonidine and ketamine can be added to optimise pain control. An intravenous lidocaine infusion can be used in challenging cases such as in opioid-dependent patients. Thoracotomies can be managed with thoracic epidural catheters which also enable earlier mobilisation. It is important to have an excellent support network surrounding the acute pain team to assist with enhanced recovery pathways and to manage pain in challenging clinical situations.

Key Points

- Pain management in intensive care is complex; it can affect outcome and hospital stay.
- An A1 (analgesia first) approach emphasises effective analgesia before sedation.
- Simple analgesics, systemic analgesics and regional blocks can be used depending on the individual patient plan and available resources.
- Delirium and complex comorbidities can make the assessment of pain difficult in intensive care patients.

References

1. Narayanan M, Venkataraju A, Jennings J. Analgesia in intensive care: part 1. *BJA Educ* 2016; 16(2): 72-8.
2. Venkataraju A, Narayanan M. Analgesia in intensive care: part 2. *BJA Educ* 2016; 16(12): 397-404.

Chapter 42

Pain management in special populations

Mahesh Kodivalasa

Pain management in a pregnant patient

- One of the most important factors to consider while prescribing medications for pregnant patients is to contemplate the effects on the foetus.
- Paracetamol has a good safety and efficacy profile in all stages of pregnancy. All basic analgesic regimens can comprise paracetamol in the management plan.
- Evidence has failed to demonstrate increased teratogenicity following therapeutic doses of NSAIDs in the first trimester of pregnancy.
- The use of NSAIDs in the final trimester can pose a risk to the foetus. NSAIDs reduce the production of prostaglandin which in turn may lead to constriction or closure of the ductus arteriosus. The consequent pulmonary hypertension can lead to foetal death.
- No links have been established between the use of opioids during pregnancy and associated teratogenicity. However, neonatal withdrawal is a known risk with long-term use of opioids in late pregnancy.
- Conditions needing the continuation of long-term opioids in pregnant patients should be a shared decision between multiple specialists with an appropriate plan in place for the delivery and neonatal care.
- Anti-neuropathic drugs have a teratogenic potential in early pregnancy. Like opioids, they can also pose a sedation risk for the newborn. The risks and benefits should be carefully weighed up for their continuation in pregnancy.

- In a breastfeeding mother, a non-opioid analgesic regimen should be the first choice to minimise the impact on maternal and infant alertness.
- Paracetamol and NSAIDs are generally safe and effective.
- If opioids are needed, the lowest effective dose should be used. Morphine is considered an ideal opioid in breastfeeding women due to the limited transfer in breast milk and poor oral bioavailability in infants.
- The Medicines and Healthcare products Regulatory Agency (MHRA), in the UK, contraindicates codeine in breastfeeding women. Dihydrocodeine or tramadol can be considered instead.
- The limited data available suggest that anti-neuropathic medications such as amitriptyline and gabapentinoids are only passed in very low amounts in breast milk, but it is sensible to monitor the child for drowsiness and other side effects especially if the mother is on a larger dose.

Pain management in a paediatric patient

- Multimodal analgesia is the ideal regimen for acute pain management.
- Non-pharmacological and non-interventional techniques such as cuddling, tactile stimulation and distraction strategies also play a significant role. The use of sucrose in neonates has been tried in procedural pain relief (Cochrane review).
- A good knowledge of various routes of administration of medications and their pharmacokinetics is very important (e.g. buccal/oral lozenges/nasal/rectal, etc.).
- Paracetamol and NSAIDs are usually sufficient for mild to moderate pain. They also have an opioid-sparing effect. Opioids are useful in the management of moderate to severe pain.
- The MHRA states that codeine should only be used to relieve acute moderate pain in children older than 12 years. It should be used only if the pain cannot be relieved by other painkillers such as paracetamol or ibuprofen. Codeine is contraindicated in all children younger than 18 years who are undergoing an adenoidectomy or tonsillectomy for obstructive sleep apnoea.

- Paediatric chronic pain is complex and challenging. This is mainly owing to the impact on the child (education, mental wellbeing and social development), on the family (social and financial impact) and on society (economic costs of medical care, social care and loss of productivity).
- Early referral to a multidisciplinary specialised paediatric pain clinic helps to achieve a better prognosis and outcome.
- Pharmacological therapies should be on a short-term trial for achieving set goals and to engage in functional recovery. Non-pharmacological and non-interventional techniques such as education, physiotherapy and psychology-based strategies are key components in the management plan. Complementary therapies have a role.
- The main aim of the multidisciplinary approach is to achieve overall functional recovery in the child.

Pain management in an elderly patient

- History taking and pain assessment can pose challenges owing to communication problems and cognitive impairment that often coexist.
- A multimodal (pharmacological, non-pharmacological and interventional) approach with an agreed realistic goal is important in managing chronic pain in the elderly.
- Non-pharmacological strategies include goal-directed physiotherapy, psychological support and complementary therapies.
- Pharmacokinetics and pharmacodynamics alter with advancing age. This is further complicated by polypharmacy and drug interactions. Elderly patients have a reduced physiological reserve and are susceptible to sedative medications.
- Paracetamol is a safe first-line treatment for the management of persistent pain, particularly of musculoskeletal origin.
- Caution should be exercised with long-term NSAIDs owing to their significant side effect profile. COX-2 inhibitors pose more cardiovascular risk. The general rule for NSAIDs is to use the lowest effective dose for the shortest time necessary.

- Opioids pose a risk of drowsiness, dizziness, confusion, and an increased incidence of falls. Side effects such as sedation, nausea and vomiting, may be worse around the time of opioid initiation or dose escalation. This may resolve after 2-3 days. Opioid-induced constipation does not readily improve and needs regular laxatives.
- Anti-neuropathic drugs are useful in the management of neuropathic pain. Drugs such as amitriptyline also help in patients with sleep disturbances. The risks should be weighed up alongside any comorbidities, drug interactions and increased sedation.
- Other drugs and routes of administration with minimal systemic effects can be explored (e.g. capsaicin cream, capsaicin patch, local anaesthetic patch, etc).

Key Points

- One of the most important factors to consider while prescribing medications for pregnant patients is to consider the effects on the foetus.
- In a breastfeeding mother, a non-opioid analgesic regimen should be the first choice to minimise the impact on maternal and infant alertness.
- The main aim of the multidisciplinary approach in managing paediatric chronic pain is to achieve functional recovery in the child.
- A multimodal approach with an agreed realistic goal is important in managing chronic pain in the elderly.

References

1.   Ray-Griffith SL, Wendel MP, Stowe ZN, Magann EF. Chronic pain during pregnancy: a review of the literature. *Int J Womens Health* 2018; 10: 153-64.

2.   Hotham N, Hotham E. Drugs in breastfeeding. *Australian Prescriber* 2015; 38(5): 156-9.

3.   Wren AA, Ross AC, D'Souza G, *et al.* Multidisciplinary pain management for pediatric patients with acute and chronic pain: a foundational treatment approach when prescribing opioids. *Children* (Basel) 2019; 6(2): 33.

4.   Stevens B, Yamada J, Ohlsson A, *et al.* Sucrose for analgesia in newborn infants undergoing painful procedures. *Cochrane Database Syst Rev* 2016; 7(7): CD001069.

5.   Reid MC, Eccleston C, Pillemer K. Management of chronic pain in older adults. *BMJ* 2015; 350: h532.

Chapter 43

Pharmacology — simple analgesics — paracetamol

Pradeep Mukund Ingle

Paracetamol is a simple analgesic and antipyretic medication. Derived from phenol, it is N-acetyl-para-aminophenol with a core benzene ring structure.

The routes of administration are: IV, PO, PR and IM.

Paracetamol doses

- The Medicines and Healthcare products Regulatory Agency (MHRA), UK, patient safety update, 2010, recommends IV infusion doses based on body weight:
  - for term newborns, infants, toddlers and children <10kg — 7.5mg/kg (maximum daily dose 30mg/kg); this was changed after multiple accidental overdose cases were reported;
  - for children weighing between 10 to 33kg — 15mg/kg (maximum daily dose 60mg/kg; without exceeding 2g);
  - for children and adults between 33 to 50kg — 15mg/kg (maximum daily dose 60mg/kg; without exceeding 3g);
  - for adolescents and adults >50kg — 15mg/kg (maximum daily dose 4g).
- Orally — 500mg to 1g every 4 to 6 hours (maximum 4g in 24 hours).
- Rectal dose — 500mg to 1g every 4 to 6 hours (maximum 4g in 24 hours).

Caution should be taken in patients weighing <50kg and the dose limited to 15mg/kg with a maximum dose of 60mg/kg in 24 hours.

Mechanism of action

The actual mechanism of action for paracetamol remains poorly understood. Several mechanisms have been postulated:

- Inhibits prostaglandin-E synthesis in the anterior hypothalamus.
- A role in the serotonergic pathway, opioid pathway, nitric oxide pathway and cannabinoid pathway.
- Inhibitor of prostaglandin synthesis in the COX pathway peripherally, and a likely peroxide-dependent mechanism (explaining a low anti-inflammatory effect).
- Central COX-3 (variant of COX-1 enzyme) inhibition.
- Blocks afferent transmission from peripheral nociceptors.

Pharmacokinetics

- Oral bioavailability is 70-90%, absorbed through the small intestine.
- Rectal bioavailability is around 40% but this varies a lot.
- Metabolised in the liver predominantly by glucoronidation (much more than sulphation) to non-toxic conjugates.
- A small amount of paracetamol undergoes cytochrome P450 system oxidisation to form N-acetyl-p-benzoquinone imine (NAPQI). This is a toxic metabolite which can cause acute liver necrosis on its accumulation. Normally, NAPQI is detoxified by glutathione conjugation to form metabolites (cysteine and mercapturic acid conjugates) which are excreted renally. However, in conditions such as glutathione deficiency or its depletion (paracetamol overdose), NAPQI can accumulate leading to hepatotoxicity. This can also cause renal and neurological issues which when combined with liver damage could be life-threatening. It is important to remember that paracetamol toxicity can also occur in a staggered manner over a period of time.
- The onset of analgesia (oral and rectal route) is 40 minutes, with a peak effect at around 1 hour.
- On IV administration the onset of action occurs in around 5 minutes with its peak occurring at 40 to 60 minutes.

- The effect of paracetamol usually lasts up to 6 hours on IV administration.
- It has a high lipid solubility and low protein binding (<20%) with a half-life of around 2.5 hours.

Adverse effects

Serious adverse effects are fortunately rare with paracetamol and it has a well-established safety profile. Also, it is safe in pregnancy and breastfeeding. Some important adverse effects include the following:

- Nausea, vomiting, bloating, dyspepsia and abdominal pain can occur sometimes.
- Can contribute to medication overuse headache.
- Transient hypotension with or without tachycardia following a rapid IV infusion of paracetamol is not uncommon.
- A possible role in the development of asthma — increasing evidence over the last two decades.
- Very rare — blood dyscrasias (thrombocytopenia, leukopenia and neutropenia) and hypersensitivity reactions (ranging from rash to anaphylactic shock).

An overdose of paracetamol in adults can cause hepatotoxicity which can begin with doses of more than 4g. With doses of more than 15g, irreversible centrilobular necrosis can occur. Nausea, vomiting and abdominal pain are the initial symptoms which may settle within 24 hours. Subsequently, symptoms of liver damage in the form of right subcostal pain and tenderness occur. Liver damage peaks 3 to 4 days after paracetamol ingestion which can lead to bleeding, low glucose levels, hepatic encephalopathy, renal damage with acidosis and cerebral oedema.

Number needed to treat (NNT)

The NNT for paracetamol in acute pain settings is 3.8. The NNT in managing cancer pain with paracetamol is 5.

Key Points

- Paracetamol is widely used and has a good safety profile and effectiveness.
- The mechanism of action is poorly understood with likely multiple central and peripheral mechanisms in place.
- Paracetamol toxicity needs to be recognised and treated immediately; the intake of more than 4g/day is associated with toxic side effects.

References

1. Analgesia — mild-to-moderate pain. Scenario: Paracetamol. London: National Institute for Health and Care Excellence, 2015. https://cks.nice.org.uk/analgesia-mild-to-moderate-pain#!scenario:1. Accessed on 16th July 2020.

2. Sharma CV, Mehta V. Paracetamol: mechanisms and updates. *Contin Educ Anaesth Crit Care Pain* 2014; 14(4): 153-8.

3. Oxberry SG, Simpson KH. Pharmacotherapy for cancer pain. *Contin Educ Anaesth Crit Care Pain* 2005; 5(6): 203-6.

Chapter 44

Pharmacology — non-steroidal anti-inflammatory drugs (NSAIDs)

Pradeep Mukund Ingle

Non-steroidal anti-inflammatory drugs (NSAIDs) are used in a variety of acute and chronic pain conditions as below:

- Mild to moderate acute pain — musculoskeletal pain, acute sprain, dysmenorrhoea, acute gout, postoperative pain and dental pain.
- Useful for their opioid-sparing effect in the management of pain.
- Management of chronic pain conditions such as arthritis and ankylosing spondylitis.
- Cancer pain conditions.
- Salicylates (low-dose aspirin) are used as antiplatelet drugs to reduce the risk of ischaemic damage in conditions such as ischaemic heart disease, strokes, TIAs, pre-eclampsia and peripheral vascular diseases.

Classification (■ Table 44.1)

Table 44.1. Classification of NSAIDs.

Group	Classes	Examples
Non-selective COX inhibitors	Salicylates	Aspirin
	Acetic acid derivatives	Diclofenac, indomethacin, ketorolac
	Fenamates	Mefenamic acid
	Oxicam derivatives	Meloxicam, piroxicam
	Propionic acid derivatives	Ibuprofen, naproxen
Selective COX-2 inhibitors	Pyrazoles	Celecoxib, parecoxib, etoricoxib

Routes of administration

The routes of administration are PO, IM, IV and PR.

There are topical applications (e.g. ibuprofen [5% and 10%] and diclofenac gels) and transdermal patches (e.g. diclofenac epolamine 1% — 140mg patch).

Cyclo-oxygenase-2 inhibitors

Cyclo-oxygenase-2 inhibitors are selective inhibitors of the COX-2 enzyme, which is an inducible enzyme. Although they have the potential advantage of fewer gastrointestinal side effects, many of them have been withdrawn from the market owing to their increased cardiovascular side effects especially with long-term use. Currently, parecoxib is commonly used in managing acute pain, especially in the postoperative period. Celecoxib and etoricoxib are two other COX-2 inhibitors in use.

Mechanism of action of NSAIDs (■ Figure 44.1)

The mechanism of action is via cyclo-oxygenase (COX) inhibition — the COX-1 and COX-2 enzymes are responsible for the synthesis of prostaglandins from membrane phospholipids. These prostaglandins cause fever, pain and an inflammatory response. NSAIDs inhibit the COX enzymes and minimise the production of these prostaglandins. Some NSAIDs are more selective than others with COX-1 and COX-2 inhibition. NSAIDs prevent the formation of prostaglandins and thromboxanes from the membrane phospholipids.

COX-1 is the constitutional form of the enzyme which mediates prostaglandin production and this is largely responsible for gastric mucosal protection, maintenance of renal blood flow and thromboxane synthesis (responsible for platelet aggregation, adhesion and vasoconstriction).

COX-2 is mainly the inducible form of the enzyme which is synthesised as a result of tissue injury and this is responsible for the production of prostaglandins (PGE2) that promotes an inflammatory response and pain in the tissue. COX-2 also mediates prostacyclin (PGI2) production which is responsible for vasodilation and inhibition of platelet aggregation.

Inhibition of prostaglandins that are produced in the central nervous system is largely responsible for the antipyretic action of NSAIDs.

There is an alternative proposed central mechanism for NSAIDs — they may block noxious inputs at the spinal level.

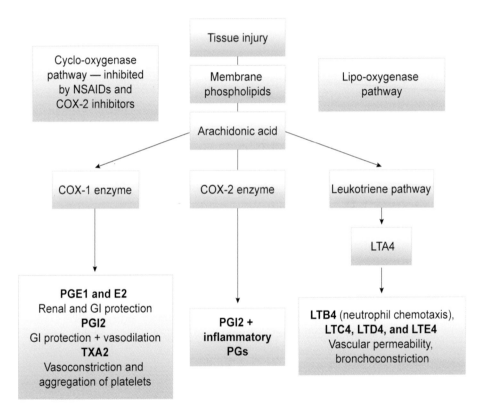

Figure 44.1. Mechanism of action of NSAIDs. COX = cyclo-oxygenase; GI = gastrointestinal; LT = leukotriene; PG = prostaglandin; PGI2 = prostacyclin; TX = thromboxane.

Salicylates

Aspirin (acetylsalicylic acid) has been used commonly to manage pain, fever and various inflammatory conditions initially. Topically, salicylic acid ointments have been used in managing pain conditions such as arthritis.

Aspirin inhibits the COX-1 and COX-2 pathways; however, in low doses it is COX-1 inhibition that predominates and this reduces prostaglandin H2 formation from arachidonic acid. This results in reduced thromboxane synthesis.

By inhibiting thromboxane A2 production (without much effect on prostacyclin production), low-dose aspirin prevents platelet aggregation and vasoconstriction. This can be used for the primary and secondary prevention of arterial thromboembolism. It is an irreversible process for the life span of platelets (7 to 14 days) and has been widely used for the prevention of atherothrombotic processes in situations such as ischaemic heart disease, the prevention and treatment of acute myocardial infarction and stroke, transient ischaemic attacks (TIAs), the prevention of vascular stent thrombosis, the prevention of vascular graft occlusions and for peripheral vascular diseases.

COX-2-mediated anti-inflammatory effects require a much larger dose compared with its antiplatelet dose (75-150mg per day).

Current guidelines in the UK consider it safe to continue aspirin peri-operatively and before anaesthetic and pain procedures, including a central neuraxial block. Concomitant administration of other anticoagulant drugs along with aspirin increases the risk of bleeding significantly.

Aspirin can cause Reye's syndrome if it is administered to treat children (<16 years age) with a recent viral infection including flu or chickenpox. Reye's syndrome is rare but a fatal complication caused secondary to the widespread mitochondrial damage eventually leading to brainstem and liver dysfunction.

Doses of aspirin in adults

- Antiplatelet dose — 75-150mg PO.
- Prevention of pre-eclampsia in at-risk women (from 12 weeks onwards) — 75-150mg PO.
- Acute ischaemic stroke and myocardial infarction — 300mg PO.
- For the management of fever and analgesia — 300-900mg 4-6 hourly PO (maximum 4g per 24 hours).
- Acute migraine — 900mg PO — single dose taken at the onset.

Pharmacokinetics

NSAIDs are rapidly absorbed in the small intestine. They are highly bound to proteins and have a low volume of distribution. Metabolism is hepatic and is followed by the excretion of inactive metabolites via urine and bile.

Adverse effects

- Renal — COX-1 and COX-2 inhibition of prostacyclin (PGI2) and prostaglandin E2 (PGE2) leads to sodium and water retention, and hypertension along with reduced glomerular filtration.
- Gastrointestinal tract — COX-1 inhibition leads to reduced PGE2 production. This can increase the risk of peptic ulcer formation and also a GI bleed (due to the loss of a protective effect from PGE2). Heavy smoking and alcohol use worsens the gastrointestinal side effects.
- Asthma can be precipitated in about 14% of asthmatics, likely due to the arachidonic acid being diverted to the leukotriene pathway.
- Cardiovascular — causes an imbalance of PGI2 and TXA2 leading to a prothrombotic state (more so with selective COX-2 inhibitors) leading to complications such as myocardial infarction and stroke.
- Can potentially affect bone healing by influencing bone formation and resorption.
- Low-dose aspirin can cause inhibition of platelet aggregation secondary to irreversible inhibition of COX-1 in platelets. Other

NSAIDs may affect platelets in a similar manner and cause an increased bleeding risk as well.
- Hepatotoxicity in an excess dose or long-term use.

Risk profile of NSAIDs

- Lowest risk — ibuprofen (renal, GI, thrombotic).
- Intermediate risk — diclofenac, naproxen, ketoprofen, piroxicam, indomethacin.
- Highest risk — azapropazone.

Contraindications

- Hypersensitivity/allergy.
- GI — symptomatic gastric or duodenal ulcers, GI bleed/perforation.
- Renal — AKI/CKD with an eGFR <30ml/min/1.73m^2.
- CVS — severe heart failure; IHD — may worsen renal function.
- Uncontrolled hypertension.
- Thrombotic conditions — cerebrovascular disease, arterial thrombotic risk; selective COX-2 inhibitors increase the risk for atherothrombotic events by about 3/1000 people/year (compared with placebo).
- Severe hepatic impairment with hypoalbuminaemia.

Cautious use

NSAIDs should be used with caution in the following:

- Elderly — increased risk of serious adverse effects — GI bleeding and perforation.
- History of peptic ulceration (standard NSAIDs contraindicated), or those at high risk of GI adverse effects.
- Inflammatory bowel disease — risk of developing or cause exacerbations of ulcerative colitis or Crohn's disease.

- Hepatitis or cholestasis — increased risk of gastrointestinal bleeding and fluid retention.
- Renal impairment (avoid if possible) — sodium and water retention leading to a deterioration in renal function.
- Heart failure and hypertension.
- In females trying to conceive.

Drug interactions of NSAIDs

- Corticosteroids — increased risk of gastric ulceration and bleeding.
- Low-dose aspirin — increases bleeding risk; use gastric protective agents.
- Angiotensin-converting enzyme (ACE) inhibitor or an angiotensin II receptor antagonist (e.g. losartan, candesartan, etc.) — increased risk of renal failure, raised blood pressure.
- Thiazide diuretics — reduced effect of diuretics.
- Loop diuretics — reduces their antihypertensive effect.
- Potassium-sparing diuretics — can cause acute kidney injury.
- Antidepressants — increased risk of upper gastrointestinal bleeding with SSRIs and SNRIs.
- Anticoagulants including newer oral anticoagulants — increased gastrointestinal bleeding risk. Avoid a combination with NSAIDs and consider gastric protection with H2 receptor antagonists or proton pump inhibitors if using for the short term.
- NSAIDs can also interact with other drugs such as cyclosporine, methotrexate, quinolones, lithium, beta-blockers (reduced efficacy), nicorandil (GI bleed) and antifungals such as fluconazole (increased NSAID levels).

Number needed to treat (NNT)

- Diclofenac 50mg — 2.7.
- Ibuprofen 200mg — 2.7.
- IM ketorolac 10mg — 2.6.
- Parecoxib 40mg IV — 2.2.

Commonly used NSAIDs

Commonly used NSAIDs and their dosages are highlighted in ■ Table 44.2.

Table 44.2. Commonly used NSAIDs and dosages.*

Drug	Route of administration	Dosage examples in adults
Ibuprofen	PO, topical	PO dose 300-400mg 3-4 times/day
Naproxen	PO	PO dose 250-500mg BD
Ketorolac	IV, IM	IV dose 10-30mg TDS
Mefenamic acid	PO	PO dose 500mg TDS
Diclofenac sodium	PO, IV, IM, topical, transdermal	PO dose 75-150mg in 2-3 divided doses
Indomethacin	PO	PO dose 150-200mg in 2 divided doses
Parecoxib	IV, deep IM	IV dose 20-40mg BD
Celecoxib	PO	PO route 100mg BD

*Please follow the BNF guidance whilst using these drugs in clinical practice.

Evidence-based trials

VIGOR (Vioxx Gastrointestinal Outcomes Research) trial

This trial compared the gastrointestinal (GI) long-term safety of rofecoxib 50mg OD vs. naproxen 500mg BD in the management of rheumatoid arthritis with a median follow-up of 9 months in patients.

The rate of confirmed GI events was significantly lower with rofecoxib as expected (2.1 vs. 4.5 events per 100 patient-years). However, the rate of serious thrombotic adverse events (myocardial infarction) was significantly higher with rofecoxib (0.4%) compared with naproxen (0.1%). The rofecoxib group had 1.67 events per 100 patient-years compared with 0.7 in the naproxen group.

APPROVe (Adenomatous Polyp Prevention On Vioxx) study

This study reported an increased cardiovascular risk of rofecoxib compared with placebo and led to the withdrawal of rofecoxib. The relative risk for a thrombotic event was 1.92.

CLASS (Celecoxib Long-term Arthritis Safety Study) trial

This trial was a randomised controlled trial in 4573 patients treated for 6 months comparing celecoxib 400mg BD vs. standard NSAIDs (ibuprofen 800mg TDS or diclofenac 75mg BD) for upper GI toxicity along with other adverse effects.

In this study, celecoxib, despite its higher than usual clinical dose, was associated with a lower incidence of symptomatic ulcers and its related complications including chronic GI bleeding, GI intolerance, liver or renal toxicity compared with NSAIDs. There was no difference in the incidence of cardiovascular events between celecoxib and NSAIDs irrespective of concomitant aspirin use for the duration of the trial.

Key Points

- NSAIDs continue to be an important class of drugs for the management of acute and chronic pain especially associated with inflammation.
- Aspirin has other important indications due to its antiplatelet actions in the prevention of atherothrombotic events.
- Beware of the renal, GI and cardiovascular side effect profile of NSAIDs before prescribing.
- The possibility of drug interactions MUST be taken into consideration while prescribing NSAIDs especially in patients on pre-existing polypharmacy.
- COX-2 inhibitors can be associated with lower GI adverse effects but at the cost of increased thrombotic effects with long-term use.

References

1. Non-steroidal anti-inflammatory drugs (NSAIDs). AnaesthesiaUK. https://www.frca.co.uk/article.aspx?articleid=101336. Accessed on 16th July 2020.

2. Bajaj S, Whiteman A, Brandner B. Transdermal drug delivery in pain management. *Contin Educ Anaesth Crit Care Pain* 2011; 11(2): 39-43.

3. Aspirin. London: National Institute for Health and Care Excellence. https://bnf.nice.org.uk/drug/aspirin.html. Accessed on 16th July 2020.

4. NSAIDs — prescribing issues. London: National Institute for Health and Care Excellence, 2019. https://cks.nice.org.uk/nsaids-prescribing-issues#!scenarioRecommendation:1. Accessed on 16th July 2020.

5. Bombardier C, Laine L, Reicin A, *et al*. Comparison of upper gastrointestinal toxicity of rofecoxib and naproxen in patients with rheumatoid arthritis. *N Engl J Med* 2000; 343: 1520-8.

6. Bresalier RS, Sandler RS, Quan H, *et al*. Cardiovascular events associated with rofecoxib in a colorectal adenoma chemoprevention trial. *N Engl J Med* 2005; 352: 1092-102.

7. Silverstein FE, Faich G, Goldstein JL, *et al*. Gastrointestinal toxicity with celecoxib vs. nonsteroidal anti-inflammatory drugs for osteoarthritis and rheumatoid arthritis: the CLASS study: a randomized controlled trial. Celecoxib Long-term Arthritis Safety Study. *JAMA* 2000; 284(10): 1247-55.

8.   Smart S, Aragola S, Hutton P. Antiplatelet agents and anaesthesia. *Contin Educ Anaesth Crit Care Pain* 2007; 7(5): 157-61.

9.   Vásquez RSV, Romero RP. Aspirin and spinal haematoma after neuraxial anaesthesia: myth or reality? *Br J Anaesth* 2015; 115(5): 688-98.

Chapter 45

Pharmacology — opioids

Rajinikanth Sundara Rajan and Pradeep Mukund Ingle

Opioid classification

Opioids can be classified into natural, semi-synthetic and synthetic derivates:

- Natural alkaloids — morphine, codeine, thebaine.
- Semi-synthetic derivatives — diacetylmorphine (heroin).
- Synthetic derivatives:
  - phenyl piperidine derivatives — pethidine, fentanyl, alfentanil;
  - cyclohexanol derivative — tramadol;
  - phenylheptylamine derivative — methadone;
  - ester derivative — remifentanil.

Opioid receptors

Endogenous opioid peptides act as ligands on different opioid receptor subtypes and produce their effects; endorphins, enkephalins, dynorphins and the recently added nociceptin orphanin FQ (N/OFQ).

The classification of opioid receptor subtypes are shown in ■ Table 45.1.

Table 45.1. The classification of opioid receptor subtypes.

Receptor subtypes	Location	Effects	Agonists/ antagonists
μ/MOP/mu	Cerebral cortex, basal ganglia, spinal cord, periaqueductal grey and peripheral tissues	Analgesia (supra-spinal and spinal), respiratory depression, constipation, nausea, vomiting, euphoria, bradycardia, pruritis, dependence, tolerance, addiction	*Agonists:* morphine, codeine, fentanyl, alfentanil, sufentanil, remifentanil, pethidine, oxycodone, methadone, endorphin, enkephalin *Antagonists:* naloxone, naltrexone, nalbuphine *Partial agonist:* buprenorphine
κ/KOP/kappa	Central nervous system	Spinal analgesia, sedation, dysphoria, meiosis	*Agonists:* morphine, dynorphin, nalorphine *Antagonists:* naloxone, naltrexone
δ/DOP/delta	Cerebral cortex, spinal cord	Spinal analgesia, respiratory depression, constipation	*Agonist:* enkephalins *Antagonist:* naloxone
N/OFQ (nociceptin orphanin FQ)	Central nervous system	Produce analgesia at high doses and hyperalgesia at lower doses	

All receptor types are linked to inhibitory G-proteins and on activation, this results in the closure of voltage gated calcium channels, hyperpolarisation by potassium efflux and adenylyl cyclase inhibition that leads to reduced cyclic adenosine monophosphate (cAMP) and a reduced release of neurotransmitters. The overall effect results in inhibition of the ascending excitatory pathway and activation of the descending inhibitory pathway. Opioids also exert an analgesic effect through activation of peripheral opioid receptors.

Pharmacology of commonly used opioids (Table ■ 45.2)

Table 45.2. Pharmacology of commonly used opioids.

	Relative lipid solubility	pKa	Volume of distribution (L/kg)	Protein bound (%)	Clearance (ml/kg/min)	Elimination half-life (min)
Morphine	1	8.0	3.5	35	16	3 hrs
Fentanyl	600	8.4	4.0	83	13	3.5 hrs
Alfentanil	90	6.5	0.6	90	6	1.6 hrs
Remifentanil	20	7.1	0.3	70	40	20 min
Pethidine	30	8.7	4.0	60	12	4 hrs

Morphine

Morphine is a weak base (pKa=8.0). When administered orally, it is absorbed in the small intestine where it is unionized. It has an oral bioavailability of 30% due to a high first pass metabolism. Peak action after an IV bolus occurs in 10 minutes.

Morphine is metabolised by glucuronidation in the liver and gut. The metabolic products are morphine 3-glucuronide and morphine 6-glucuronide. Morphine is also demethylated to normorphine. Morphine 6-glucuronide is more potent than the parent compound. Morphine 3-glucuronide and normorphine are inactive. It is excreted by the kidneys and bile. Morphine 6-glucuronide accumulates in renal failure.

Pharmacodynamics of morphine:

- Cardiovascular system — hypotension and bradycardia with histamine release.
- Respiratory system — respiratory depression, a reduced response to CO_2 but the response to hypoxia is less affected, bronchospasm and suppression of cough response. With a poor lipid solubility there is a risk of delayed respiratory depression with intrathecal/epidural administration. It can be used as an antitussive.
- Gastrointestinal and genitourinary systems — sphincter of Oddi contraction, and urinary retention as a result of an increased detrusor and sphincteric tone.
- Endocrine system — reduces ACTH, prolactin and gonadotrophic hormones; increases ADH secretion.

Diamorphine

Diamorphine is diacetyl morphine, a prodrug and is around twice as potent as morphine. It has a high lipid solubility, enabling it to be administered subcutaneously (2.5-5mg 4-hourly). It has less of a risk of delayed respiratory depression. It is metabolised by ester hydrolysis to mono-acetyl morphine and morphine.

Codeine

Codeine is 3-methyl morphine, a prodrug and is classed as a weak opioid. Codeine undergoes less first pass metabolism than morphine. Codeine is metabolised mostly by glucuronidation. It undergoes N-demethylation to nor-codeine. Around 10% undergoes O-demethylation to morphine, that has a significant analgesic effect. O-demethylation is influenced by cytochrome P450 (CYP2D6). CYP2D6 is absent in 9% of Caucasians, which results in poor analgesia.

Dihydrocodeine

Dihydrocodeine is around twice as potent as codeine. Metabolism of dihydrocodeine is also influenced by CYP2D6.

Fentanyl

Fentanyl is a selective μ agonist with a rapid onset of action and is 100 times more potent than morphine. Transdermal fentanyl is available at 12μg/hr, 25μg/hr, 50μg/hr and 100μg/hr, the dose is titrated clinically, and is used sparingly in chronic pain rather than acute pain as a steady-state plasma equilibrium is delayed for 18-24 hours. Buccal, intranasal and sublingual preparations are used for breakthrough pain in patients with chronic cancer pain.

Fentanyl has a high lipid solubility (600 times that of morphine). At lower doses (1-2μg/kg), it is rapidly redistributed (13 minutes). Higher doses and intravenous infusion have a variable elimination half-life. It is demethylated to nor-fentanyl, an inactive compound. Fentanyl can cause chest wall rigidity and bronchospasm.

Alfentanil

Alfentanil has one fifth the potency of fentanyl. It has a lower lipid solubility and has a rapid onset of action, because 90% is unionized at a pH of 7.4. It has a smaller volume of distribution contributing to a shorter elimination half-life, despite smaller clearance.

Remifentanil

Remifentanil is a derivative of fentanyl with a similar potency. Remifentanil is rapidly metabolised by non-specific esterases to inactive compounds, resulting in a shorter elimination half-life. Its duration of action is not influenced by hepatic and renal dysfunction. Unlike other opioids, remifentanil's context sensitivity half-life is not affected by the duration of infusion. Side effects include bradycardia, hypotension and chest wall rigidity. Hyperalgesia is reported to occur with prolonged intravenous infusions.

Pethidine

Pethidine has one tenth the potency of morphine. Pethidine has a 50% oral bioavailability and is metabolised in the liver by phase 1 reactions. One of the metabolites, nor-pethidine, has a longer half-life (14-21 hours) and accumulates in renal dysfunction. Pethidine has serious interactions with mono-amine oxidase inhibitors (MAOIs) due to serotonergic hyperactivity and causes cardiovascular instability, convulsions and coma. It also has anticholinergic effects.

Tramadol

Tramadol is a racemic mixture of two stereoisomers. One exerts analgesia through μ-agonism and a reduced neuronal reuptake of serotonin. Another isomer inhibits the reuptake of noradrenaline modulating the descending inhibitory pathway.

Tramadol is metabolised in the liver. One of the metabolites may accumulate in patients with renal dysfunction. Tramadol has a similar efficacy and potency to pethidine. It causes less respiratory depression and constipation, but can cause convulsions. It can interact with tricyclic antidepressants and selective serotonin reuptake inhibitors resulting in serotonergic hyperactivity.

Oxycodone

Oxycodone is a semi-synthetic derivative of thebaine. It is a μ-agonist with the same analgesic efficacy as morphine. Oxycodone has nearly twice the oral bioavailability as morphine. It is metabolised by N-demethylation to noroxycodone and O-demethylation to normorphine. Normorphine has a strong analgesic activity. Oxycodone should be avoided if the eGFR is less than 10ml/min.

Methadone

Methadone is a synthetic opioid, commonly used in cancer pain and opioid abuse patients. It is a μ-receptor agonist and NMDA receptor antagonist. Methadone has a high and variable bioavailability (35-100%). It is 89% protein bound and has a longer half-life (20-35 hours). It is metabolised in the liver and excreted in urine and faeces. 25-50% is excreted unchanged renally. At higher doses, methadone is known to cause Q-T prolongation and torsades de pointes.

The peri-operative management of patients on methadone is complex and should be done by specialists involving the acute pain team.

Tapentadol

Tapentadol is a novel drug with dual actions; it acts as an opioid agonist and inhibits the reuptake of noradrenaline. It has the same analgesic efficacy as oxycodone. Tapentadol can induce seizures and should be cautiously used in a known epileptic. It is reported to cause serotonergic syndrome when coadministered with drugs such as tricyclic antidepressants, selective serotonin reuptake inhibitors (SSRIs) and serotonin-norepinephrine reuptake inhibitors (SNRIs).

Opioid partial agonists

Opioid partial agonists have a limited effect on μ-receptors. They have a ceiling effect on analgesia and side effects such as respiratory depression. Increasing the dose beyond the maximal effect does not yield additional effects. Examples of partial agonists are:

- Buprenorphine is a semi-synthetic opioid. It acts as an agonist at the μ-receptor, an antagonist at the κ-receptor and an agonist at the N/OFQ receptor. It exerts analgesia at low doses and has an anti-analgesia effect at higher doses. It is more potent than morphine and has a longer duration of action (10 hours) due to a high receptor affinity. It is commonly administered as a transdermal application. It is available in a sublingual tablet and solution for injection.

- Nalorphine is a partial agonist and is used as an antagonist.

Mixed agonists-antagonists

Mixed agonists-antagonists, such as pentazocine and nalbuphine, act as an antagonist at the μ-receptors and an agonist at the κ-receptors.

μ-receptor antagonists

Naloxone has the highest affinity for μ-receptors compared with other opioid receptors. It reverses the analgesic effect and other opioid effects such as respiratory depression and pruritis. It is the drug of choice in opioid overdosage. It can be carefully titrated to effect, and thus offset respiratory depression and preserve analgesia. Naloxone can cause pulmonary oedema, hypertension and cardiac arrhythmias and anti-analgesia in opioid-naïve patients. Naloxone has a shorter duration of action (30-40 minutes).

Naltrexone has a similar action to naloxone. It has a higher oral bioavailability than naloxone and has a longer half-life (24 hours).

Key Points

- Opioids are classified into natural, semi-synthetic and synthetic.
- Opioid receptor subtypes include MOP, KOP, DOP and N/OFQ.

References

1. Rowbotham D, Macintyre P. *Clinical pain management: acute pain*. Arnold Publishers, 2003.

2. McDonald J, Lambert DG. Opioid receptors. *Contin Educ Anaesth Crit Care Pain* 2015; 15(5): 219-24.

3. Azzam AAH, McDonald J, Lambert DG. Hot topics in opioid pharmacology: mixed and biased opioids. *Br J Anaesth* 2019: 122(6): e136-45.

Chapter 46

Problems of opioid use in chronic pain

Thanthullu Vasu

Opioids can become a problem rather than a solution in chronic pain; although they are very good analgesics for acute pain, there is little evidence for long-term use. The Faculty of Pain Medicine, UK, has created a guideline — *Opioids Aware*. It clarifies that the initiation, tapering or stopping of opioids should be made in agreement with the patient, general practitioner and all members of the healthcare team.

In those whom it helps, opioids should be used in a low dose and used intermittently; the proportion of patients where it helps is very small and it is difficult to identify this at the start. The risk of opioid harm increases substantially at doses of more than 120mg morphine equivalent per day.

Pain clinics should be open and honest while discussing this; if opioids do not help, they should be stopped, even if no other treatment is available. If a trial of 2-4 weeks has not helped, the patient should be weaned off the drug and it stopped altogether.

An appropriate detailed assessment including the assessment of emotional aspects are vital before considering opioids in chronic pain. If these medications are started, regular reviews with an assessment of emotional status is important. It is ideal to have a single prescriber, usually the general practitioner who can assess and give prescriptions for short durations if needed.

Long-term use harms

Endocrine system

The hypothalamic-pituitary-adrenal axis and the gonadal system can be inhibited by opioids in the long term. Hypogonadism can lead to problems in both sexes (infertility, reduced libido, amenorrhoea, depression, etc).

Fractures and falls

Opioids increase the risk of falls and associated fractures (relative risk of 1.38). Bone density reduction has been observed with long-term opioid use.

Immune system

Opioids can induce immunosuppression due to their effects on immune effector cells and action on the central nervous system.

Opioid-induced hyperalgesia

The prolonged use of opioids can itself cause hyperalgesia due to changes in neuroplasticity; the mechanisms proposed include:

- Central glutaminergic system, NMDA system.
- Increase in spinal dynorphins.
- Spinal nociceptive processing neuron activation.
- Genetic mechanisms.
- Decreased uptake of neurotransmitters from primary afferents.

Pain in this condition can be more diffuse than pre-existing pain. Treatment includes reducing the opioid dose gradually or by opioid rotation.

Key Points

- *Opioids Aware* from the Faculty of Pain Medicine is a useful educational tool.
- More than 120mg/d of morphine equivalent should be alarming and referral to a multidisciplinary pain service is vital.
- If an opioid trial does not help a patient in 2-4 weeks, it should be stopped.
- Long-term harms include their effect on the hormonal system, immunological system and bones.
- Opioid-induced hyperalgesia can cause diffuse pain; it needs to be recognised and opioid reduction or rotation is essential.

References

1. Opioids Aware. Faculty of Pain Medicine of the Royal College of Anaesthetists. https://www.fpm.ac.uk/opioids-aware. Accessed on 16th July 2020.

2. Seyfried O, Hester J. Opioids and the immune system. *Br J Pain* 2012; 6: 17-24.

Chapter 47

Pharmacology — gabapentinoids

Pradeep Mukund Ingle

Pregabalin was launched around 2004 in the UK whereas gabapentin has been in use a few years prior to this. They have been used widely in the management of neuropathic pain across the world.

The indications are as follows:

- Neuropathic pain.
- Anticonvulsant.
- Generalised anxiety disorder (GAD) — as a second-line medication as per the NICE guidelines.

Off-label use in conditions such as fibromyalgia, migraine, pain conditions other than neuropathic pain, mania and bipolar conditions, and alcohol abuse is not uncommon.

These drugs are also increasingly being used as adjuvant drugs to manage peri-operative analgesia. In acute peri-operative pain, there is good evidence for a reduction in postoperative pain (level 1 evidence) with reduced opioid consumption. There is also some evidence for gabapentinoids being helpful in the prevention of chronic post-surgical pain and functional improvement in post-surgical patients.

In patients with chronic pain they are commonly used in managing conditions such as post-herpetic neuralgia, pain from spinal cord injury, painful diabetic peripheral neuropathy, and neuropathic/mixed cancer pain.

Doses in chronic pain

The route of administration for pregabalin and gabapentin is oral. For managing pain in adults, pregabalin can be started from 75mg BD and gradually increased up to a maximum of 300mg BD as tolerated. In adults, gabapentin is started at a dose of 300mg on day 1, increased to 300mg BD on day 2, followed by establishing a dose of 300mg TDS from day 3 onwards. This dose is gradually increased as tolerated by 300mg increments every 2 to 3 days up to a maximum dose of 1.2g TDS. In the elderly and people at risk of developing dose-related adverse effects, doses as low as 100mg can be used to start with and escalation of the dose will need to be at a slower rate. After a trial of 6 to 8 weeks, if it is not found to be beneficial for pain, gabapentin will need to be weaned off gradually. In a similar way, pregabalin can be started at 25mg BD in the elderly and at-risk patients.

Mechanism of action

Multiple mechanisms have been proposed.

Gabapentinoids bind to the α2-δ1 subunit of voltage gated calcium channels leading to a reduction of pre-synaptic calcium influx, thereby reducing excitatory neurotransmitter release (such as glutamate, substance P, CGRP). They reduce the neurotransmitter release in neuronal tissues.

Gabapentinoids also reduce the sensitivity of the dorsal horns of the spinal cord through multiple mechanisms and stimulate the uptake of glutamate by excitatory amino acid transporters.

Other actions at the dorsal horn can include inhibition of descending serotonergic pathways along with stimulation of descending inhibitory pathways.

Presynaptic plasticity is mediated through thrombospondins (astrocyte-derived glycoproteins). Gabapentin may block the binding between thrombospondin and α2-δ1 subunits which in turn can inhibit the generation of excitatory synapses.

Besides this, gabapentinoids can alter the affective response to pain by suppression of areas in the pre-frontal cortex, which has connections with the limbic system.

There is limited evidence for their actions on NMDA receptors, sodium channels and their anti-inflammatory action (inhibition of pro-inflammatory cytokines).

Their anxiolytic and sleep-modulating effects make them suitable adjuvants in managing acute pain situations such as peri-operative pain.

Pharmacokinetics

Pregabalin is two to three times more potent as an analgesic compared with gabapentin. Pregabalin has a better pharmacokinetic profile in terms of rapid absorption, it is predictable and has a better bioavailability orally. It also has a longer duration of action.

Adverse effects

Pregabalin

Sedation, dizziness, somnolence, vomiting, visual disturbances (generally transient), increased appetite, weight gain, GI side effects such as a dry mouth, constipation, flatulence, nervous system disorders such as ataxia, tremor, vertigo, and lethargy along with central nervous system side effects such as confusion, mood changes, disorientation and, rarely, suicidal ideation.

Gabapentin

Gabapentin has a similar risk profile in addition to other reported adverse effects such as leukopenia and respiratory issues including respiratory depression, dyspnoea and an increased risk of infections and pneumonia.

Drug interactions

Gabapentinoids may cause potentiate sedation if used in combination with other CNS depressants such as lorazepam and ethanol.

Both gabapentin and pregabalin are not recommended in pregnancy and breastfeeding patients.

Setting realistic expectations with gabapentinoids at the start of prescription and informing patients about the need to wean them down, should they not be helpful for the pain condition, is important.

Regular reviews are essential to assess the benefits and risks of prescription along with any evidence for abuse, dependence, addiction, misuse and drug diversion.

Number needed to treat

The number needed to treat ranges between 4.2 to 6.4.

Gabapentinoid abuse

Gabapentinoid prescriptions increased by 50% between 2011 to 2013. In the year 2016, approximately 12 million prescriptions were issued for gabapentinoids in the UK.

The risk of increasing abuse is concerning; pregabalin is more likely to be abused compared with gabapentin. The UK government has reclassified gabapentinoids as class C controlled drugs from April 2019 under the Misuse of Drugs Act 1971. It is now an offence to unlawfully possess, supply (or intent to supply) or even allow the premises for its unlawful use.

Withdrawal symptoms usually begin 24-48 hours after the cessation of gabapentinoids. These include craving, nausea, insomnia, anxiety, agitation, tremors, generalised pains, excessive sweating, an inability to focus, hypertension and convulsions in severe cases. In addition to the above, headache, nervousness, dizziness, depression, diarrhoea and flu-like syndrome can occur with pregabalin withdrawal.

Suggested gradual weaning rates are a 50-100mg daily dose per week for pregabalin and 300mg every 4 days for gabapentin by Public Health England (PHE).

Key Points

- Gabapentinoids are increasingly used in chronic pain management.
- They need to be trialled for a sufficient duration (weeks) before assessing their effectiveness and suitability in pain management.
- Their limitations need to be understood by doctors prescribing them to minimise their unwanted effects and abuse.
- With their rising use, abuse has become a growing concern which needs a structured approach in order to support these patients.

References

1. Ramaswamy S, Wilson JA, Colvin L. Non-opioid-based adjuvant analgesia in perioperative care. *Contin Educ Anaesth Crit Care Pain* 2013; 13(5): 152-7.

2. Fallon MT. Neuropathic pain in cancer. *Br J Anaesth* 2013; 111(1): 105-11.

3. Neuropathic pain — drug treatment. Pregabalin. London: National Institute for Health and Care Excellence, 2020. https://cks.nice.org.uk/neuropathic-pain-drug-treatment#!prescribingInfoSub:5. Accessed on 16th July 2020.

4. Neuropathic pain — drug treatment. Gabapentin. London: National Institute for Health and Care Excellence, 2020. https://cks.nice.org.uk/neuropathic-pain-drug-treatment#!prescribingInfoSub:12. Accessed on 16th July 2020.

5. Chincholkar M. Analgesic mechanisms of gabapentinoids and effects in experimental pain models: a narrative review. *Br J Anaesth* 2018; 120(6): 1315e-34.

6.   Ingle P, Murally H, Sundararajan R, *et al*. Anonymous survey of gabapentinoids in patients attending the chronic pain service at a university hospital in Staffordshire in the United Kingdom. *Br J Pain* 2020; 14(2) Supplement 15-36: 18-9.

7.   Advice for prescribers on the risk of the misuse of pregabalin and gabapentin. Public Health England. https://assets.publishing.service.gov.uk/government/uploads/system/uploads/attachment_data/file/385791/PHE-NHS_England_pregabalin_and_gabapentin_advice_Dec_2014.pdf. Accessed on 17th July 2020.

8.   Parson G. Guide to the management of gabapentinoid misuse. https://www.prescriber.co.uk/article/guide-to-the-management-of-gabapentinoid-misuse. Accessed on 17th July 2020.

9.   Ozturk HM, Morkavuk G. Nasal pregabalin overdose and myclonus: a new way of misuse. *Psychiat Clin Psych* 2019; 29(2): 216-9.

10.   Evoy KE, Morrison MD, Saklad SR. Abuse and misuse of pregabalin and gabapentin. *Drugs* 2017; 77: 403-26.

Chapter 48

Pharmacology — other anti-neuropathic agents

Harnarine Murally and Pradeep Mukund Ingle

The main classes of drugs used to manage neuropathic pain are antidepressants and anticonvulsants. These include:

- Tricyclic antidepressants (TCAs) such as amitriptyline and nortriptyline.
- Serotonin norepinephrine reuptake inhibitors (SNRIs) such as duloxetine and venlafaxine.
- Anticonvulsants — gabapentinoids, phenytoin, carbamazepine and lamotrigine. (Please refer to Chapter 47, Pharmacology — gabapentinoids.)

Tricyclic antidepressants

These are first-line drugs for the management of neuropathic pain in accordance with the NICE guidelines. Nortriptyline is reported to have fewer side effects than amitriptyline and is recommended in the elderly, but it is more expensive than amitriptyline. The number needed to treat (NNT) is 3.6.

The route of administration is oral.

Mechanism of action

Tricyclic antidepressants inhibit presynaptic noradrenaline and serotonin reuptake (see ■ Table 48.1 on p258).

Pharmacokinetics

Tricyclic antidepressants are well absorbed in the gut due to their high lipid solubility. They have an extensive first pass metabolism, are highly protein bound and have a large volume of distribution. They are metabolised in the liver with active metabolites which are excreted via the kidneys (see ■ Table 48.2 on p259).

Side effects

- Due to anticholinergic properties — dry mouth, constipation, blurred vision, urinary retention.
- Antihistamine — drowsiness, increased gastric pH.
- Alpha-adrenoceptor blockade — orthostatic hypotension; a quinidine-like effect — prolonged QT interval, atrioventricular block and torsades de pointes.

Contraindications

Arrhythmias, during the manic phase of bipolar disorder, heart block, immediately post-myocardial infarction.

Pregnancy and breastfeeding

Tricyclic antidepressants should only be used in pregnancy if the benefit outweighs the risk.

They are safe to use whilst breastfeeding (minimal amounts are secreted in the breast milk).

Drug interactions

- MAOIs and bupropion — increased risk of severe toxic reaction; levodopa — decreases absorption of levodopa.

- Lithium — potentially increases the risk of neurotoxicity.
- Fluoxetine and paroxetine — an increased risk of toxicity and hyponatraemia.
- Thiopental — an increased risk of arrhythmias and hypotension.

Withdrawal

Withdrawal of the drug occurs within 5 days of stopping and usually symptoms are mild but they can be severe in some patients. It should be tapered gradually over 2-4 weeks.

Duloxetine (SNRI)

Duloxetine is one of the first-line drugs for managing neuropathic pain. It is administered orally and has a NNT of 6.4

Mechanism of action

Duloxetine inhibits presynaptic noradrenaline and serotonin reuptake equally (see ■ Table 48.1).

Pharmacokinetics

Please refer to ■ Table 48.2.

Pregnancy and breastfeeding

There is a risk of neonatal withdrawal if near term. Duloxetine should only be used if the benefit outweighs the risk. It is delivered in breast milk, hence, it is best avoided.

Drug interactions

Warfarin, DOACs, heparin, aspirin and alteplase — increased risk of bleeding.

Venlafaxine (SNRI)

Venlafaxine is used as a second-line drug in the treatment of neuropathic pain. Venlafaxine achieves analgesic effects over 4-6 weeks. It is taken orally and has a NNT of 6.5.

Mechanism of action

Venlafaxine inhibits only presynaptic serotonin reuptake at doses less than 150mg/day. There is some effect on noradrenaline reuptake at higher doses (see ■ Table 48.1).

Table 48.1. Mechanism of action and side effects of antidepressant neuropathic drugs.

Drug	Noradrenaline reuptake inhibition	Serotonin reuptake inhibition	Sedation	Anti-muscarinic activity	Orthostatic hypotension
Amitriptyline	++	++++	High	High	Moderate
Nortriptyline	++	+++	Moderate	Moderate	Low
Duloxetine	++	++	Low	Low	Low
Venlafaxine	+	+++	Low	Low	Low

Table 48.2. Pharmacokinetics of antidepressant neuropathic drugs.

Drug	Dose mg	Bioavailability %	Protein binding %	Half-life Hours
Amitriptyline	10-75	30-60	96	30-40
Nortriptyline	10-75	30-80	92	18-44
Duloxetine	30-120	50	95	12
Venlafaxine	75-225	45	30	5-11

Anticonvulsants

Carbamazepine

Carbamazepine is the first-line drug in the treatment of trigeminal neuralgia. It can be given via oral and rectal routes. Due to white cell count changes, blood test monitoring is needed. The usual dose is 300-800mg/d in three divided doses but the maximum dose is 1200mg/d.

Mechanism of action

A voltage gated sodium channel blocker.

Pharmacokinetics (see ■ Table 48.3)

Carbamazepine induces hepatic enzymes which reduces its own half-life with a repeated dosage.

Common side effects

Drowsiness, dizziness, headaches and migraines, impaired motor coordination, constipation, nausea and vomiting.

Serious side effects

Agranulocytosis, drug-induced hepatitis, Stevens-Johnson syndrome.

Pregnancy

Teratogenic — causes facial abnormalities, IUGR, microcephaly and mental retardation.

Oxcarbazepine

Oxcarbazepine is a keto-analogue of carbamazepine and does not pass through liver cytochrome metabolism; this results in an improved side-effect profile and fewer drug interactions. It is better tolerated than carbamazepine. It is started at 150mg twice daily and is increased gradually up to maximum of 1800mg/d.

Lamotrigine

Lamotrigine is used as a second-line drug to treat HIV polyneuropathy, trigeminal neuralgia, post-stroke pain and painful diabetic neuropathy.

Mechanism of action

It blocks voltage activated sodium channels. It also reduces the effects of the excitatory neurotransmitter, glutamate.

Pharmacokinetics (see ■ Table 28.3)

It is metabolised in the liver by glucuronidation and exhibits 'autoinduction' similar to carbamazepine.

Common side effects

Vomiting, dizziness, drowsiness, headache, diplopia, ataxia and confusion.

Serious side effects

A rash which can progress to Stevens-Johnson syndrome and toxic epidermal necrolysis, liver problems.

Phenytoin

Phenytoin is used in the treatment of trigeminal neuralgia. It is not a first-line drug for treating neuropathic pain. It can be given intravenously in an acute attack. The dose is tailored to each patient as wide inter-patient variability exists. Approximately 10% of the population is a slow hydroxylator.

Mechanism of action

Phenytoin blocks Na^+ channels and reduces Ca^{2+} entry leading to enhanced GABA activity.

Pharmacokinetics

It demonstrates saturable hepatic hydroxylation resulting in zero-order kinetics just above the therapeutic range (see ■ Table 28.3).

Table 48.3. Pharmacokinetics of anticonvulsants.

Drug	Dose mg	Bioavailability %	Protein binding %	Half-life Hours
Phenytoin	200-600	90	90	22
Carbamazepine	200-1200	100	75	16-36
Lamotrigine	25-400	98	56	24

Common side effects

Nausea, stomach pain, loss of appetite, poor coordination, hirsutism, acne, gum hyperplasia.

Serious side effects

Drowsiness, self-harm, liver problems, bone marrow suppression, low blood pressure and toxic epidermal necrolysis.

Pregnancy

Phenytoin is teratogenic (craniofacial abnormalities and mental retardation).

Drug interactions

Phenytoin induces hepatic mixed function oxidases which increase the metabolism of warfarin, benzodiazepines and the oral contraceptive pill.

Key Points

- Tricyclic antidepressants are cheap and are first-line neuropathic medications. The NNT is 3.6. A dry mouth is a common side effect and caution must be exercised if the patient has an arrhythmia.
- Duloxetine is a first-line anti-neuropathic drug (SNRI). The NNT is 6.4.
- Carbamazepine and oxcarbazepine are first-line drugs for trigeminal neuralgia.

References

1. Finnerup NB, Attal N, Haroutounian S, *et al.* Pharmacotherapy for neuropathic pain in adults: systematic review, meta-analysis and updated NeuPSIG recommendations. *Lancet Neurol* 2015; 14(2): 162-73.

2. Colloca L, Ludman T, Bouhassira D, *et al.* Neuropathic pain. *Nat Rev Dis Primers* 2017; 3: 17002.

Chapter 49

Pharmacology — local anaesthetics

Vanja Srbljak and Pradeep Mukund Ingle

Local anaesthetics (LAs) are a diverse group of drugs that reversibly block the sensation of pain in body areas where they are administered. They can be applied topically, administered intrathecally, epidurally, intravenously or they can be infiltrated within the vicinity of peripheral nerves depending on the drug.

Mechanism of action

They act by reversibly blocking the voltage gated sodium (Na⁺) channels of nerve fibres. Suppressing the action potential inhibits the transmission of

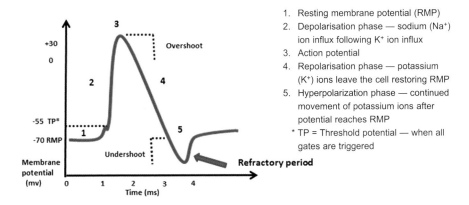

1. Resting membrane potential (RMP)
2. Depolarisation phase — sodium (Na⁺) ion influx following K⁺ ion influx
3. Action potential
4. Repolarisation phase — potassium (K⁺) ions leave the cell restoring RMP
5. Hyperpolarization phase — continued movement of potassium ions after potential reaches RMP
* TP = Threshold potential — when all gates are triggered

Figure 49.1. Action potential phases of a neuron.

nerve impulses further (■ Figure 49.1). Impulse conduction becomes interrupted when a critical length of a nerve fibre is blocked.

Classification

Local anaesthetics (LAs) are divided into two different classes based on their chemical structure:

- Esters — contain para-aminobenzoic acid (PABA).
- Amide local anaesthetics — without PABA.

Structural components of local anaesthetics

The structural component of LAs include an aromatic ring (usually substituted), intermediary chain and ionizable amino group.

Factors influencing the activity of a LA (■ Table 49.1)

- Lipophilic aromatic group — determines lipid solubility, potency, nerve penetration, onset time and duration.
- Intermediary link — categorizes the type of the LA. It is more potent if the intermediate chain is longer, e.g. bupivacaine is three times more potent than lignocaine.
- Hydrophilic amine group — confers water solubility and a LA's precipitation.
- Protein binding — determines the duration of action and is a predictor of LA toxicity.
- pKa (the pH at which 50% of the drug is ionized and 50% is present as a base) — a lower pKa means that more of the unionised fraction is present for any given pH and consequently the faster the onset of action will be.

Table 49.1. Pharmacokinetic determinants of local anaesthetics.

Factor	Action
Lipid solubility	Determines the onset of action
Protein binding	Determines the duration of action
pKa	Determines the speed of action

- Route of administration — systemic absorption of an LA varies with the route of administration. Absorption from the lowest to highest: subcutaneous injection < brachial plexus < epidural route < caudal < intercostal blocks and topical anaesthesia. Absorption of LAs is influenced also by the dosage, use of epinephrine, characteristics of drugs and the mode of administration.
- Intrinsic properties of LAs — they can exhibit vasodilator (e.g. lignocaine and bupivacaine at low doses) and vasoconstrictor properties (e.g. cocaine) which can affect their absorption.

Metabolism

Ester-based LAs are metabolised rapidly by plasma pseudo-cholinesterase, hence they have a short half-life (except cocaine, hydrolysed in the liver).

Amide-based LAs are metabolised by liver amidases in the liver via CP450 enzymes (prilocaine is metabolised extra-hepatically in the lungs). They have a longer half-life and acitivity.

Physicochemical characteristics of local anaesthetics are outlined in ■ Table 49.2 overleaf.

Table 49.2. Comparison table for physicochemical characteristics of local anaesthetics.

Agent	pK	Protein binding %	Potency	Recommended max dose mg/kg	Relative duration (hours)	Toxicity	Partition coefficient at 36°C	Vd l/kg	t½ min
Esters									
Procaine	8.9	6	1	12	1	Low	3.1	0.7	9
Chloroprocaine	8.7	Low	4	11	45 min	Low	17	0.3	1
Tetracaine	8.5	76	16	1-3	1.5	Medium	541	1	8
Amides									
Lidocaine	7.9	64	1	3-7*	1-2	Medium	110	1	100
Prilocaine	7.9	55	1	6-9*	1.5	Low	50	1.9	261
Ropivacaine	8.1	94	4	3	3-12	Medium	230	0.8	110
Bupivacaine	8.1	95	4	2	3-12	Medium	560	1	60
Levobupivacaine	8.1	97	4	2	3-12	Medium	27.5	1	60

* Higher range figure is for likely safe doses of LAs with adrenaline (insufficient data).

Adverse reactions

- Toxicity. Local toxicity is usually a localised allergic reaction (mostly secondary to PABA), myotoxicity, neurotoxicity, transient neurological symptoms (associated mostly with 2-5% intrathecally administered lidocaine). Intra-articular LAs can cause chondrotoxicity. Systemic toxicity is associated with neurological and cardiovascular features:
  - CNS — an initial excitatory state followed by a depressive phase. Manifests usually as peri-oral tingling, tinnitus together with slurred speech, lightheadedness and tremor, confusion or

agitation progressing to generalized convulsions with coma and respiratory depression;

- CVS — myocardial depression, bradycardia, hypotension, arrhythmias leading to cardiac arrest.

The management of LA systemic toxicity is in accordance with the Association of Anaesthetists of Great Britain and Ireland (AAGBI) guidelines.

- Methaemoglobinaemia (due to the accumulation of o-toluidine) can shift the oxy-haemoglobin dissociation curve to the left and reduce the ability of haemoglobin to release oxygen to the tissues. Prilocaine, benzocaine and lidocaine can cause methaemoglobinaemia.

- Allergic reactions. The amide type LAs can cause localised hypersensitivity reactions. Anaphylaxis is an uncommon complication mainly related to preservatives in the LA (e.g. methylparaben) or with an ester type LA.

Commonly used local anaesthetics

- Amethocaine (tetracaine) is available as a 4% cream and topical conjunctival preparation. It is the least metabolised of the ester LAs and hence possesses a higher risk of toxicity.

- Lidocaine is the most widely used local anaesthetic drug. The maximum recommended doses are 3mg/kg without adrenaline and 7mg/kg with adrenaline.

- Ropivacaine is available as a levo-rotatory stereoisomer of propyl derivate, making it less cardiotoxic compared with racemic mixtures of other local anaesthetics. It has motor block sparing properties in lower concentrations.

- Bupivacaine exists as a racemic mixture of enantiomers. It is the longest acting local anaesthetic and is cardiotoxic on IV administration. The maximum recommended dose is 2mg/kg. It is three to four times more potent than lidocaine, but its onset of action is much slower.

- Levobupivacaine is the S-enantiomer of bupivacaine. It has less CNS toxicity, CVS toxicity and a lesser vasodilatatory effect compared with bupivacaine.
- EMLA cream is the eutectic mixture of 2.5% prilocaine and 2.5% lignocaine. The melting point of this mixture is below room temperature making it possible to penetrate the skin more easily. Both components are in an unionized state in EMLA cream and ionisation occurs only after absorption.

Additives for local anaesthetics

- Dextrose — added to bupivacaine to increase the density of the solution. This increases the specific gravity of bupivacaine to 1.026 at 20°C, making it hyperbaric comparing with cerebrospinal fluid.
- Epinephrine (adrenaline) — adding adrenaline to local anaesthetics increases the duration of nerve blockade, decreases systemic toxicity and reduces surgical bleeding. Its concentration is usually between 1:80,000 (common in dental practice with 2% lignocaine), 1:200,000 (most common in solutions of LAs) and 1:400.000 (2.5µg/ml). The maximum safe dose of adrenaline should be limited to 200µg over 10 minutes or 300µg over 1 hour.
- Felypressin — a vasoconstrictor derived from vasopressin, is used as an adjunct to lidocaine and prilocaine to prolong their action.
- Hyaluronidase — used to improve the speed of onset of local anaesthetic blocks (e.g. in eye surgeries) as it increases membrane permeability.
- Carbonation of LAs — increases the proportion of the non-ionised drug and hence it penetrates nerve cell membranes more rapidly. Alkalinisation of LA solutions can have a similar effect.

Key Points

- Local anaesthetics reversibly prevent pain by interrupting nerve conduction.
- The typical structure of LAs consists of the hydrophilic tertiary amine and hydrophobic aromatic ring. The linking between these groups determines the pharmacological properties of the LA.
- LAs are safe medications to use with a long tradition but they can cause systemic and local adverse reactions.
- Additives can improve the analgesic properties of local anaesthetics.

References

1. Taylor A, McLeod G. The mechanism of local anaesthetics on voltage gated sodium channels and other ion channels. *Br J Anaesth* 2002; 89(1): 52-61.

2. Taylor A, McLeod F. Basic pharmacology of local anaesthetics. *BJA Educ* 2020; 20(2): 34-41.

3. Webb ST, Ghosh S. Intra-articular bupivacaine: potentially chondrotoxic? *Br J Anaesth* 2009; 102(4): 439-41.

4. Management of severe local anaesthetic toxicity. Association of Anaesthetists, 2010. https://anaesthetists.org/Home/Resources-publications/Guidelines/Management-of-severe-local-anaesthetic-toxicity. Accessed on 20th July 2020.

5. Barash M, Reich K, Rademaker D. Lidocaine-induced methemoglobinemia: a clinical reminder. *J Am Osteopath Assoc* 2015; 115: 94-8.

6. Christie LE, Picard J, Weinberg GL. Local anaesthetic systemic toxicity. *BJA Educ* 2015; 15(3): 136-42.

7. Whiteman A, Bajaj S, Hasan M. Novel techniques of local anaesthetic infiltration. *Contin Educ Anaesth Crit Care Pain* 2011; 11(5): 167-71.

8. Neill S. Local anaesthetics. AnaesthesiaUK. https://www.frca.co.uk/SectionContents.aspx?sectionid=235. Accessed on 20th July 2020.

9. Marri SR. Adjuvant agents in regional anaesthesia. *Anaesth Intensive Care Med* 2015; 16(11): 570-3.

Chapter 50

Pharmacology — topical agents

Ashok Puttappa and Pradeep Mukund Ingle

Topical preparations act as 'targeted' peripheral analgesics for localised neuropathic and nociceptive pain. They have an advantage over systemic drugs as their pharmacological action is mainly by local activity in the nerves and peripheral tissues with clinically insignificant serum levels. However, some drugs such as topical opioid patches do not act locally but are used for their advantage of a steady systemic release over long periods.

Topical agents/patches with a localised peripheral action

Lignocaine 5% patch

An adhesive plaster (10 x 14cm) containing 700mg lignocaine (equivalent to 5% w/w).

Mechanism of action

* Sodium channel blocker.
* Inhibits the expression of nitric oxide and pro-inflammatory cytokines from T cells which is helpful in inflammatory conditions.

Application

Lignocaine patches are applied over painful areas for not more than a 12-hour period in 24 hours (typically a 12-hour 'on' and 12-hour 'off' schedule). Note: one should not apply more than three patches at a time. Two to four-week regular applications are needed to obtain maximal benefit.

Uses

Lignocaine patches are licensed for neuropathic pain due to post-herpetic neuralgia (PHN). However, they have also been used in peripheral neuropathic pain other than PHN and inflammatory arthritis, especially osteoarthritis. The NNT is 4.4.

Side effects

Application site burning, pruritus, dermatitis, rash and, rarely, headache.

Cautious use

Severe hepatic disease and in patients on anti-arrhythmic drugs.

Capsaicin

Capsaicin is trans-8-methyl-N-vanillyl-6-nonenamide, a component of red chilli pepper. It is available as a cream or lotion (0.025% and 0.075%) and as a patch.

The capsaicin patch (Qutenza®) 8% measuring 14cm x 20cm (280cm^2 patch) contains 179mg capsaicin or 640µg of capsaicin per cm^2.

Mechanism of action

Various mechanisms have been proposed for its effects:

- Substance P depletion from presynaptic terminals depresses type C nociceptive fibre function.
- Neurodegeneration by reducing the growth of pain-related epidermal nerve fibres.

Application

Capsaicin cream should be applied three to four times per day over intact, non-inflamed skin. A time gap of at least 4 hours should be maintained between two successive applications.

A capsaicin patch must be applied by a qualified healthcare worker. It is applied over intact, non-irritated, dry skin only. The patch remains in place for 30 minutes for the feet and 60 minutes for other locations and removed subsequently. It may be repeated every 90 days if pain returns. It is licensed for diabetic and non-diabetic peripheral neuropathic pain.

Uses

Neuropathic pain due to post-herpetic neuralgia, painful diabetic neuropathy, persistent post-surgical pain (post-thoracic surgeries/post-mastectomy chronic pain), osteoarthritis and rheumatoid arthritis. The NNT is 6.7.

Side effects

Pain and erythema at the application site (very common), pruritus, papules, vesicles, inflammation, dryness at the application site (common), burns, sneezing and coughing on inhalation.

Eutectic mixture of local anaesthetics (EMLA)

Composition — lignocaine 2.5% + prilocaine 2.5%.

Mechanism of action

Absolute sodium channel blockade of sensory nerves causing dense anaesthesia (compared with lignocaine which causes a less dense effect).

Uses

Post-herpetic neuralgia, postoperative pain (acute/chronic), before IV cannulation (apply 1 hour before the procedure).

Side effects

Pallor, erythema, itching, rash and rarely methaemoglobinaemia.

Amethocaine (Ametop® gel)

Composition — 4% tetracaine.

Mechanism of action

It acts by blocking sodium channels in line with other local anaesthetics.

Uses

It is used for topical application before IV cannulation similar to EMLA cream. However, it has an advantage of an early onset (30-45 minutes) with its effects lasting up to 6 hours.

Side effects

Local histamine and serotonin release can cause erythema and local oedema in some patients.

Topical NSAIDs

Available for various NSAIDs, e.g. diclofenac, ibuprofen (5% and 10%).

Uses

Osteoarthritis and chronic musculoskeletal pain.

NNT — topical diclofenac 9.3, topical ketorolac 6.4.

Side effects

Itchiness, rash (rare).

Topical nitrates (e.g. nitroglycerin ointment and patches)

Mechanism of action

Stimulates ATP-sensitive K$^+$ channels (increased cGMP).

Uses

Tendinopathies (tennis elbow), osteoarthritis and chest pain. They are applied for 12 hours in a 24-hour period.

Side effects

Headache.

Topical analgesic patches for systemic action

Transdermal drug delivery

Delivery of the medicine to the general circulation occurs through the skin surface in these drugs. These drugs need to have a low molecular weight and high lipid solubility for better absorption. Absorption occurs through diffusion with a high concentration gradient in the delivery system and zero concentration in the skin.

The advantages are:

- No oral intake is required, which avoids first pass inactivation by the liver.
- Controlled absorption, resulting in a uniform plasma concentration.

The disadvantages are:

- Skin irritation or sensitivity may occur.
- This formulation is not suitable for many drugs and it may be an expensive option with certain drugs.
- A risk of unreliable absorption in patients with poor circulation, e.g. patients in circulatory shock.

- Exposure to excess direct heat (e.g. peri-operative warming mattress) or sunlight can increase the absorption of opioids transdermally resulting in an overdose.

Types of patches are a reservoir patch and matrix (drug adhesive) patch.

The components of a transdermal patch are an outermost impermeable backing layer, a reservoir holding the medication, a rate-controlling membrane, adhesive to hold the patch and lastly a peelable protective cover applied to the skin.

Buprenorphine patch

Buprenorphine is a partial μ-receptor agonist (μ agonist but κ and δ antagonist). A buprenorphine patch is a matrix type of patch and there are two types based on the duration of action — 4 days for a TransTec® patch and 7 days for a BuTrans® patch.

The BuTrans® patch is available from 5μg/hr to 20μg/hr strength in 5μg increments.

The TransTec® patch is available in 35, 52.5 and 70μg/hr strengths.

10mg oral morphine is equivalent to 5μg/hr of a buprenorphine patch.

Application

BuTrans® is applied on non-irritated, clean skin continuously up to 7 days and TransTec® up to 4 days.

Uses

Moderate to severe chronic cancer pain in opioid-naïve patients, and chronic nociceptive pain not responding to non-opioids.

Nausea, dizziness, constipation, pruritus, somnolence, dry mouth, burning, irritation at the applied site.

Fentanyl patch

Fentanyl is a µ agonist. Fentanyl patches are available in both reservoir and matrix forms of patches. Each patch maintains its plasma concentration for up to 72 hours with a peak between 12-24 hours. They have a narrow therapeutic window.

Their elimination half-life can be delayed by interaction with CYP3A4 inhibitors, such as ketoconazole, clarithromycin and amiodarone.

Starting fentanyl patches in opioid-naïve patients should be avoided. Their long-term use in the management of chronic non-cancer pain has been discouraged in view of recent evidence of significant harm from long-term opioids.

They are available as 12.5, 25, 37.5, 50, 75 and 100µg/hr strengths.

25mg/h of fentanyl is approximately equivalent to 90mg of oral morphine per day.

Uses

Moderate to severe chronic cancer pain, and severe non-cancer nociceptive pain.

Fentanyl HCl iontophoretic transdermal system (fentanyl ITS)

This is a needle-free iontophoretic PCA system which extends a transdermal system in acute pain management. In this system, ionized drug molecules are driven by electric current across the skin into the systemic circulation. Pre-programmed settings for this are 40µg per dose over 10 minutes and not more than 6 doses per hour. It functions up to 24 hours (maximum 80 doses).

The advantages over a regular patch include:

- Precise control over analgesic dose and frequency.
- Useful for acute situations such as acute postoperative pain.

Key Points

- Although topical application of analgesics is more commonly used for their local and targeted effects, they can also be used as systemic release patches for their slow sustained effects.
- Topical analgesics with local effects have minimal systemic side effects and hence they are a treatment option for those who are unable to tolerate systemic side effects of oral analgesics.
- Whilst using opioid patches one needs to be aware of their limitations which can increase or decrease their absorption in the systemic circulation thereby having less effect or delivering an overdose, respectively.

References

1. Saito I, Koshino T, Nakashima K, *et al.* Increased cellular infiltrate in inflammatory synovia of osteoarthritic knees. *Osteoarthritis Cartilage* 2002; 10: 156-62.

2. Power I. Fentanyl HCl iontophoretic transdermal system (ITS): clinical application of iontophoretic technology in the management of acute postoperative pain. *Br J Anaesth* 2007; 98(1): 4-11.

3. Bajaj S, Whiteman A, Brandner B. Transdermal drug delivery in pain management. *Contin Educ Anaesth Critical Care Pain* 2011; 11(2): 39-43.

4. https://www.medicines.org.uk/emc/product/573/smpc. Accessed on 20th July 2020.

5. https://www.medicines.org.uk/emc/product/290/smpc. Accessed on 20th July 2020.

6. Scheindlin S. Transdermal drug delivery: past, present, future. *Mol Interven* 2004; 4(6): 308-12.

7. https://www.medicines.org.uk/emc/product/794/smpc. Accessed on 20th July 2020.

8. Stow PJ, Glynn CJ, Minor B. EMLA cream in the treatment of post-herpetic neuralgia: efficacy and pharmacokinetic profile. *Pain* 1989; 39: 301-5.

9. Derry S, Conaghan P, Da Silva JAP. Topical NSAIDs for chronic musculoskeletal pain in adults. *Cochrane Database Syst Rev* 2016; 4(4): CD007400.

Chapter 51

Pharmacology — steroids

Mahesh Kodivalasa

Mechanism of action

- The primary mechanism of action of steroids is at the cellular level.
- Steroids bind to intracellular receptors, alter gene expression and regulate cellular processes.
- Inflammatory mediators play a key role in peripheral and central sensitization. Steroids inhibit the action of phospholipase and thus reduce/suppress the conversion of essential fatty acids to arachidonic acid (the precursor for inflammatory mediators such as prostaglandins and leukotrienes).
- Alteration of chemotactic activity affects the function of lymphocytes.
- IL-1 and TNF are inflammatory neurochemicals responsible for central sensitization. Steroids inhibit the expression of IL-1 and TNF which play a key role in chemotaxis, production of inflammatory mediators and cell-mediated immunity.
- Alteration of ion transport affects vascular permeability and inter-compartmental fluid shifts.
- Steroids also alter carbohydrate, protein and fat metabolism. The effects include gluconeogenesis, increased protein catabolism and redistribution of body fat. The metabolic effects also include bone catabolism and consequent osteoporosis.

A comparison of commonly used steroids is shown in ■ Table 51.1.

Table 51.1. A comparison of commonly used steroids.

Agent	Relative gluco-corticoid activity	Relative mineralo-corticoid activity	Plasma half-life (and duration of action)	Equivalent dose (comparative)
Hydrocortisone	1	1	90 min (8-12 hr)	20mg
Prednisolone	4	0.8	200 min (12-36 hr)	5mg
Methylprednisolone	5	Minimal	180 min (12-36 hr)	4mg
Triamcinolone	5	0	300 min (12-36 hr)	4mg
Dexamethasone	30	Minimal	100-300 min (36-72 hr)	0.75mg

Adverse effects associated with steroids

- Osteoporosis, fractures and osteonecrosis — steroids have been shown to stimulate osteoclastic activity and suppress osteoblastic activity.
- Adrenocortical suppression — the duration and dosage of steroids are not reliable predictors, but longer-acting formulations tend to be associated with a higher risk of adrenocortical suppression.
- Cardiovascular disease — long-term steroid therapy is known to be associated with a higher CVS risk (HTN and new onset AF).
- The risk of peptic ulcer increases significantly when used in combination with non-steroidal anti-inflammatory drugs (NSAIDs).
- Cataracts and glaucoma — the risk of both cataracts and glaucoma is increased. Although the risk is dose dependent, the individual susceptibility varies.
- Gluconeogenesis leads to poor control of diabetes.
- Potential immunosuppression can lead to a susceptibility for infections. (The Faculty of Pain Medicine — Royal College of Anaesthetists — issued a statement on steroids during the COVID-19 pandemic; see Chapter 55 for details.)

The use of corticosteroids for neuraxial procedures

The key points from the consensus statement of the British Pain Society/Faculty of Pain Medicine (Royal College of Anaesthetists) on the use of corticosteroids for neuraxial procedures in the United Kingdom are as follows:

- Particulate steroids must not be used for transforaminal cervical epidural injections on the basis of the risk of rare but catastrophic complications.
- Whilst definitive recommendations cannot be given for the choice of soluble or particulate steroid for injections in interlaminar cervical epidurals, clinicians should be aware that serious neurological complications can still occur.
- Whilst definitive recommendations cannot be given for the choice of soluble or particulate steroid for injections in epidurals undertaken in other areas of the spine (thoracic, lumbar and caudal), clinicians should be aware that serious neurological complications can occur with any route of administration particularly if there is a history of previous spinal surgery.
- Steroid preparations for epidural administration may carry a small risk of neurotoxicity with inadvertent intrathecal injection due to the preservative preparation used. The clinician should carefully consider the formulation used.
- The consent process should include discussion and documentation regarding indications, efficacy, safety and alternative treatments.

Key Points

- Steroids suppress the synthesis of inflammatory mediators, reduce chemotaxis and inhibit the expression of cytokines, such as IL-1 and TNF, which play a key role in peripheral and central pain modulation.
- The short-term and long-term potential advantages and adverse effects of steroids on individual patients should be carefully weighed up.

Chapter 52

Pharmacology of other medications — alpha-2 agonists, NMDA antagonists, muscle relaxants and others

Mahesh Kodivalasa

Alpha-2 agonists: clonidine

Clonidine is a centrally acting alpha-2 agonist.

The anti-nociceptive action is thought to be from modulation of descending noradrenergic inhibition (in the spinal cord), augmentation of endogenous opiate release and also from inhibition of sodium channels.

Clonidine has a role in both acute and chronic pain management. As an adjuvant in regional analgesia, clonidine prolongs the duration of analgesia. It is also shown to have a preventive analgesic action.

Clonidine acting synergistically with opioids could reduce overall opioid requirements. One of the newfound interests for clonidine is due to its role in the management of opioid and alcohol withdrawal symptoms in dependent patients.

It is useful as a third-line drug in intractable cancer pain management.

In addition to its availability in oral and injectable forms, clonidine is also available as a topical transdermal patch.

Clonidine has a 100% bioavailability after oral administration. It has a high lipid solubility with predominant hepatic metabolism and renal excretion.

Caution should be exercised in patients on beta-blockers or with conduction abnormalities.

NMDA antagonists: ketamine

Ketamine has non-competitive antagonistic action at the NMDA receptors.

Other actions that are thought to play a role in analgesia include: a reduction of presynaptic glutamate release (reducing calcium influx), interaction with opioid receptors and a local anaesthesia-like action by blocking sodium channels.

Ketamine has a role in both acute and chronic pain management. It has been shown to potentiate the analgesic effect of opioids while also reducing the overall dose in the peri-operative period. Ketamine has an inhibitory effect on the wind-up pain mechanism due to temporal summation (central sensitization). It can help in the multimodal management of difficult and challenging chronic pain scenarios.

A low-dose ketamine infusion in the peri-operative period has been shown to have a preventive analgesic effect. One of the other reasons for this newfound interest in ketamine in the peri-operative period is its role in the pain management of opioid-dependent and tolerant patients.

NMDA receptors play a key role in central sensitization and maintenance of a chronic pain state. Ketamine with its NMDA receptor antagonistic activity helps as an adjuvant in the management of chronic (neuropathic) pain.

Ketamine is also useful as a third-line drug in intractable cancer pain management.

NMDA receptors play a key role in the development of opioid-induced hyperalgesia (with chronic opioid usage). Ketamine's NMDA receptor antagonistic action is shown to play a beneficial role.

In addition to its most commonly available form as a liquid for systemic administration, oral administration is also possible as a solution and capsules (not easily available in the UK).

Ketamine has a 25% bioavailability after oral administration. It has a high lipid solubility with predominant hepatic metabolism and renal excretion.

The long-term use of ketamine can lead to addiction akin to opioids.

Muscle relaxants

Baclofen

Baclofen is a chemical analogue of GABA. It inhibits the pre-synaptic release of excitatory neurotransmitters (glutamate and aspartate). Its post-synaptic action involves potentiation of potassium conductance leading to membrane hyperpolarisation.

Baclofen can be administered orally and intrathecally (implantable pumps). The dose needs to be carefully adjusted in the elderly and in patients with renal failure. Cumulative doses and a synergetic action with other sedatives can be problematic. Abrupt withdrawal can lead to a severe hyperactive state, rhabdomyolysis and autonomic dysfunction.

Botulinum toxin

The main proposed action of botulinum toxin is by the inhibition of release of acetylcholine. It is available in a powder form to be diluted for immediate administration as an injection. In addition to its role in managing muscle spasms, Botox is also licensed by NICE (UK) and the FDA (USA) for the treatment of migraine headaches. Thirty-one standard spots are injected as per a NICE algorithm for migraine if standard treatments (at least three medications) have not helped and if there are more than 15 headache days per month. Botox has a good safety profile.

Benzodiazepines

Benzodiazepines bind to and modulate GABA receptors. They increase the frequency of opening of chloride channels and hyperpolarise neuronal membranes. They also inhibit the release of excitatory neurotransmitters.

The main adverse effects include sedation and dizziness. Cumulative doses and synergetic action with other sedatives and analgesics can be dangerous.

Long-term use can be addictive.

Key Points

- Alpha agonists, NMDA antagonists and muscle relaxants can be helpful in the multimodal management of difficult and challenging chronic pain scenarios.
- Ketamine has an inhibitory effect on the wind-up pain mechanism due to temporal summation (central sensitization).
- Botox is licensed by NICE guidelines for the treatment of migraines if standard treatments have not helped.

References

1. Chaparro LE, Smith SA, Moore RA, *et al.* Pharmacotherapy for the prevention of chronic pain after surgery in adults. *Cochrane Database Syst Rev* 2013; 7: CD008307.
2. Tsui PY, Chu M. Ketamine: an old drug revitalized in pain medicine. *BJA Educ* 2017; 17(3): 84-7.

Chapter 53

National guidelines in chronic pain

Thanthullu Vasu

Below is a brief summary of a few national and international guidelines; for the details, please refer to the web links provided for the full version.

NICE low back pain guideline
Low back pain and sciatica in over 16s: assessment and management
NG 59, 2016
www.nice.org.uk/guidance/ng59

Assessment of low back pain and sciatica:

- Exclude other diagnoses (red flags).
- Risk stratification (STarT Back tool).
- Do not routinely offer imaging.

Non-invasive treatments:

- Self-management.
- Group exercise programme.
- Do not offer belts/corsets/orthotics/traction.
- Do not offer acupuncture or TENS.
- Consider CBT psychology or a combined physical and psychological programme.
- Facilitate a return to work or normal daily activities.
- Do not offer paracetamol alone or opioids or SNRIs or anticonvulsants.

- NSAIDs should be used only at their lowest effective dose for the shortest period of time with gastric protection.

Invasive treatments:

- Do not offer spinal injections.
- Radiofrequency denervation if other treatments do not help and patients have moderate or severe pain, after a diagnostic block.
- Consider an epidural if there is acute and severe sciatica (not in stenosis claudication pain).
- Do not offer spinal fusion or disc replacement.
- Spinal decompression should be offered only if sciatica has not responded to treatment.

NICE headache guideline
Headaches in over 12s: diagnosis and management
CG 150, 2012 (updated 2015)
www.nice.org.uk/guidance/cg150

Assessment:

- Further investigations/referral in need.
- Red flags — a need for investigation.
- Use a headache diary (8 weeks) for a primary headache diagnosis.

Diagnosis:

- Tension-type headache, migraine, cluster headache — based on clinical features.
- Migraine with aura (aura lasting 5-60 minutes, fully reversible).
- Menstrual-related migraine — 2 days before and 3 days after periods, at least 2 of 3 cycles consecutively.
- Medication overuse headache — medications for 3 months or more.

Treatment:

- All headaches — diary, diagnosis, investigations if needed.

- Tension-type:
  - aspirin, paracetamol or NSAID for acute treatment;
  - prophylaxis — acupuncture (10 sessions over 5-8 weeks).
- Migraine:
  - acute — combination of oral triptan and NSAID/paracetamol (nasal triptan if 12-17 years old); consider antiemetics;
  - prophylaxis — topiramate or propranolol; can consider amitriptyline; consider acupuncture.
- Menstrual-related migraine — if not settled, think of frovatriptan/zolmitriptan.
- Migraine in pregnancy — paracetamol, discuss triptan/NSAID with risks.
- Cluster headache:
  - acute — oxygen +/or nasal triptan;
  - prophylaxis — verapamil.
- Medication overuse — stop for at least 1 month, stop abruptly.

NICE neuropathic pain guideline
Neuropathic pain in adults: pharmacological management in non-specialist settings
CG 173, 2013 (updated 2019)
www.nice.org.uk/guidance/cg173

Key principles:

- Agree a plan, look for a cause, coping, non-pharmacological treatments.

Treatment:

- There is a choice of amitriptyline, duloxetine, gabapentin or pregabalin (all except trigeminal neuralgia).
- Initial treatment not effective — offer one of the others.
- Tramadol should only be used for acute rescue therapy.
- Capsaicin cream for localised neuropathic pain.
- Trigeminal neuralgia — carbamazepine as the initial drug.

British Pain Society — Guidelines for pain management programmes for adults, 2013
https://www.britishpainsociety.org/static/uploads/resourc es/files/pmp2013_main_FINAL_v6.pdf

- There is good evidence for the use of cognitive behavioural Pmps as a package.
- Cost-effective, and reduce healthcare consumption.
- Promotes behaviour change and well-being.
- Standard PMP — twelve half-day sessions, a total of 36 hours.
- Longer programmes provide a greater, enduring benefit.
- Very disabled and distressed patients will need a longer programme (15-20 full days).
- Three groups — targeted early PMP, standard PMP, and intensive PMP.

NICE chronic pain guideline
Chronic pain: assessment and management
NG 10069 (in development at the time of press)
www.nice.org.uk/guidance/indevelopment/gid-ng10069

This guideline is still in development at the time of publication of this book.

NICE chronic fatigue syndrome guideline
Chronic fatigue syndrome/myalgic encephalomyelitis: diagnosis and management
CG 53, 2007
www.nice.org.uk/guidance/CG53

- Clinical diagnosis, exclude other causes.
- Duration for diagnosis — 4 months in adult, 3 months in a young person.
- Sleep management, rest periods (limit to 30 minutes), relaxation, pacing, diet, education.
- Cognitive behavioural therapy (CBT) and/or graded exercise therapy (GET).

NICE spinal cord stimulation guideline
Spinal cord stimulation for chronic pain of neuropathic or ischaemic origin
Technology appraisal guidance TA 159, 2008
www.nice.org.uk/guidance/ta159

- Recommended for chronic neuropathic pain VAS >50mm, for at least 6 months despite medications, and if a trial of stimulation is successful.
- Not recommended for pain of an ischaemic origin.
- A multidisciplinary team assessment and management are needed.

The Faculty of Pain Medicine opioid guideline
Opioids Aware
www.fpm.ac.uk/opioids-aware

This is a resource for patients and healthcare professionals for the use of opioids for pain, with five key messages:

- Very good for acute pain, but there is little evidence for long-term pain.
- A small proportion might benefit, if the dose is kept low and use is intermittent.
- The risks of harm increases if >120mg day oral morphine equivalent.
- If opioids are of no help, they should be stopped, even if there is no other treatment available.
- A very detailed assessment of emotional influences is essential.

NICE guideline on cannabis-based medicinal products
Cannabis-based medicinal products
NG 144, Nov 2019
www.nice.org.uk/guidance/ng144

- Chronic pain — do NOT offer a cannabinoid.

- Chemotherapy-induced intractable nausea and vomiting — nabilone can be an add-on treatment.
- Spasticity — 4-week trial of tetrahydrocannabinol spray in multiple sclerosis spasticity.
- Severe treatment-resistant epilepsy — research recommended.

The Faculty of Pain Medicine — Position statement on the medicinal use of cannabinoids in pain medicine, Nov 2019
https://www.fpm.ac.uk/sites/fpm/files/documents/2019-12/FPM-Cannabis-statement-2019-final_0.pdf

- The Faculty supports NICE guidance NG 144.
- The safety and efficacy are not established; we need robust trials and a database for proper analysis.
- They may have potential but a strong evidence base is needed.
- A Cochrane review in 2018 concluded there is a lack of good evidence for cannabis products.
- *Reviews in Pain* concluded that they are unlikely to be highly effective in chronic non-cancer pain.
- National reports from the USA, Australia and Ireland comment on the lack of good quality evidence.

The Faculty of Pain Medicine — Statement on cannabis clinics, March 2019
https://www.rcoa.ac.uk/news/faculty-pain-medicine-responds-establishment-independent-cannabinoid-clinics

- The Faculty is deeply concerned.
- There are very limited data on cannabinoids in pain management.
- There are concerns that clinics are introducing their use before the research by NICE is published.

SIGN chronic pain guideline
Scottish Intercollegiate Guidelines Network (SIGN)
Management of chronic pain
SIGN 136, 2013
https://www.sign.ac.uk/assets/sign136.pdf

- Assessment and planning.
- Supported self-management.
- Pharmacological management.
- Psychologically based interventions (evidence level C).
- Exercise (evidence level B).
- Advice to stay active (evidence level A).

The Faculty of Pain Medicine and British Pain Society — Outcome measures, Jan 2019
https://www.britishpainsociety.org/static/uploads/resourc
es/files/Outcome_Measures_January_2019.pdf

- Several domains — pain quantity, interference, physical functioning, emotional functioning, quality of life, patient reported global rating.
- If looking for one scale, EuroQol (EQ5D-5L) — requires a temporary user agreement. There are five dimensions: mobility, self-care, usual activities, pain/discomfort and anxiety/depression.

British Geriatrics Society
The assessment of pain in older people: UK National Guidelines, 2018
Age and Ageing 2018; 47(1): i1-i22

- Pain prevalence increases with age up to 85 years and then decreases.
- A multidisciplinary approach is required, with an assessment of cognitive ability and socio-cultural factors to be considered.
- Patient self-reporting is the most valid and reliable indicator of pain.

- Mild to moderate cognitive impairment — a numerical rating scale or verbal descriptors.
- Severe cognitive impairment — PAINAD and Doloplus-2 scales.
- The Abbey Pain Scale is widely used, but there has been no recent evaluation.

Royal College of Physicians, UK — CRPS guideline
Complex regional pain syndrome in adults — UK guidelines for diagnosis, referral and management in primary and secondary care, 2018
www.rcplondon.ac.uk/guidelines-policy/complex-regional-pain-syndrome-adults

- Diagnosis — Budapest criteria (at least two sign and three symptom categories).
- Individual chapters for specialties to manage CRPS.
- Education and reassurance.
- Neuromodulation can be used if the patient has not responded to treatment.
- Psychological interventions.

American College of Rheumatology (ACR): preliminary diagnostic criteria for fibromyalgia, 2010
Wolfe F, Clauw DJ, Fitzcharles MA, *et al*. *Arthritis Care Res* 2010; 62(5): 600-10

- Widespread Pain Index (WPI) — 19 body areas, score 0-19.
- Symptom Severity Score (SS) — fatigue, waking unrefreshed, cognitive symptoms, somatic symptoms — each scored 0-3, making a total possible score of 12.
- WPI ≥7 and SS ≥5.
- WPI 3-6 and SS ≥9.

EULAR recommendations for fibromyalgia
European League Against Rheumatism (EULAR) revised recommendations for the management of fibromyalgia, 2017
www.ard.bmj.com/content/76/2/318

- Weak evidence for — amitriptyline, pregabalin, duloxetine, acupuncture, CBT, hydrotherapy.
- Weak evidence against — NSAIDs, SSRIs, chiropractice, massage.
- Strong evidence for — exercise.
- Strong evidence against — guided imagery, homeopathy.

British Pain Society — Spinal cord stimulation for the management of pain: recommendations for best clinical practice, 2009
https://www.britishpainsociety.org/static/uploads/resourc es/files/book_scs_main_1.pdf

- Randomised controlled trials support the use of spinal cord stimulation (SCS) in failed back surgery syndrome, complex regional pain syndrome, neuropathic pain and ischaemic pain.
- The commonest infection is *Staphylococcus aureus*; patients should be screened for MRSA.
- Compatibilty with MRI scanners can be a problem.

British Pain Society — Intrathecal drug delivery for the management of pain and spasticity in adults: recommendations for best clinical practice, 2015
https://www.britishpainsociety.org/static/uploads/resources /files/itdd_2015_pro_v3.pdf

- Intrathecal drug delivery is indicated in chronic non-malignant pain (CNMP), pain in cancer and in spasticity.
- Ziconotide in CNMP has been studied.
- Opioids in CNMP — long-term concerns include tolerance, granuloma formation and hormone suppression.

- Intrathecal baclofen in cerebral and spinal spasticity.

British Pain Society and Faculty of Pain Medicine — Standards of good practice for spinal interventional procedures in pain medicine, 2015
https://www.britishpainsociety.org/static/uploads/resources/files/spinal_intervention_A5_Final_April_2015_1.pdf

- Consent, identification, environment, assistance, fluoroscopy, infection control.
- Risk assessment for anticoagulation and sedation.
- Record keeping, discharge/follow-up.

Royal College of Anaesthetists — Guidelines for provision of anaesthesia services for inpatient pain management, 2020 Chapter 11, Guidelines for the provision of anaesthesia services (GPAS)
https://www.rcoa.ac.uk/sites/default/files/documents/2020-02/GPAS-2020-11-Pain.pdf

- Staffing requirements for inpatient pain services (IPS).
- Equipment and facilities.
- Special requirements, e.g. children, emergency department, etc.
- Training and education.
- Organisation, audit, patient information.

British Pain Society and Faculty of Pain Medicine — Standards of good practice for medial branch block injections and radiofrequency denervation for low back pain, 2014
https://www.britishpainsociety.org/static/uploads/resources/files/mbb_2013_-_FINAL.pdf

- Consent, identification, environment, assistance, fluoroscopy, infection control.

- Risk assessment for anticoagulation and sedation.
- Record keeping, discharge/follow-up.

The Faculty of Pain Medicine — The good pain medicine specialist
Standards for revalidation of specialists in pain medicine, Apr 2018
https://fpm.ac.uk/sites/fpm/files/documents/2019-08/Good%20Pain%20Specialist%202018.pdf

- Knowledge, skills and performance.
- Safety and quality.
- Communications and teamwork.
- Maintaining trust.

The Faculty of Pain Medicine — Conducting quality consultations in pain medicine, May 2018
https://fpm.ac.uk/sites/fpm/files/documents/2019-08/Conducting%20Quality%20Consultations%202018.pdf

- Provide a good standard of care to your patients.
- Adequately assess the patient.
- Communicate effectively.
- Strive to adopt a shared decision-making approach.
- Formulate an individualised management plan based on the best available evidence.
- Justify a patient's trust and trust in the profession.
- Keep your patients safe.
- Provide adequate documentation.

Chapter 54

Guidance for primary care clinicians

Mahesh Kodivalasa, Gopi Boora and Uday Idukallu

Chronic pain accounts for approximately a fifth of general practice appointments. Primary care physicians are often the first point of contact for patients with chronic pain. Understanding the complexity and needs of chronic pain patients enables the delivery of patient-centred care. In the UK, societies and governing bodies such as the British Pain Society, Faculty of Pain Medicine and Royal College of General Practitioners work closely to achieve this.

It is important that primary care physicians have an adequate education and awareness about common chronic pain conditions and the associated red flags. The initial approach taken by a primary care physician should be a holistic and biopsychosocial approach. This comprises general advice and prescription. Further assessment, advice and guidance from the secondary care pain service should be readily accessible. Pain services need to be prioritised in the same way as other long-term conditions.

General practitioners should have a knowledge of local pain services (including highly specialised pain services) and their referral process. The referral process should include information on pain, current management, comorbidities and referral to other specialties especially in those patients with red flags. A close and robust communication should be reciprocated by the secondary care specialist pain service. The communication should include exchange of information regarding clinical impression, ongoing care, escalation plans, de-escalation advice and discharge plans. The emphasis should be on functional recovery with an improvement in quality of life as the main outcome goal. This should be continued in the primary care setting as well.

Shared care pathways can help to manage most patients with complex chronic pain. This will also aid to minimise the dependence on acute and emergency secondary care services. The specialist teams may include a pain service, de-addiction service, palliative service, rehabilitation service, etc.

A primary care chronic pain management service comprises primary care physicians, nurse practitioners/prescribers, community physiotherapists, psychologists, pharmacists and social care workers. It is imperative that a regular review of progress of patients with chronic pain occurs to ensure effective treatment. This helps to reduce the risk of dependence and long-term side effects. Good practice also includes safe and cost-effective prescribing.

Current local guidelines, national guidelines and safety practices (e.g. *Opioids Aware*) should be followed in prescribing and continuing medications. Knowledge regarding the various groups of medications, their mechanism of action, side effects and drug interactions would be of immense help.

Key Points

- It is important that primary care physicians have an adequate education and awareness regarding common chronic pain conditions.
- A close working relationship with a secondary care specialist pain service will enable the delivery of patient-centred care.

References

1. Scott LJ, Kesten JM, Bache K, *et al.* Evaluation of a primary care-based opioid and pain review service: a mixed-methods evaluation in two GP practices in England. *Br J Gen Pract* 2020; 70 (691): e111-9.

2. Kennedy MC, Henman MC, Cousins G. General practitioners and chronic non-malignant pain management in older patients: a qualitative study. *Pharmacy* (Basel) 2016; 4(1): 15.

3. Pain Management Services: planning for the future — guiding clinicians in their engagement with commissioners. Faculty of Pain Medicine. https://www.accs.ac.uk/document-store/pain-management-services-planning-the-future-guiding-clinicians-their-engagement. Accessed on 20th July 2020.

Chapter 55

Pain management in difficult times (COVID-19)

Thanthullu Vasu

Difficult times require a flexible and innovative working pattern from pain clinicians and their team. The COVID-19 pandemic has transformed the landscape in which pain clinicians work and so we need to plan for managing acute situations followed by the restoration of services in a calm manner. The Faculty of Pain Medicine, UK, has published guidelines to deal with such difficult situations in a timely manner.

While the pandemic placed a substantial demand on the healthcare system, most pain clinicians were redeployed to other services. It has to be remembered that patients with chronic pain can face significant distress including psychological distress during these difficult times due to a lack of interventions that control their pain. Various challenges that a pain clinician can face are outlined below.

Triage for pain services

Pain services should consider a triage system where patients are unsuitable for remote consultations. These patients might be those with complex needs, where examination is required, where medical records are unavailable and where there are issues with a patient's mental capacity and ability to process information.

Consultations with patients

The use of remote consultations (including telephone, web-based platforms) should be considered, while the safety of face-to-face consultations should be planned with the appropriate protection. Challenging situations, such as during the current pandemic, can provide opportunities to innovate pain services and use innovative technologies.

The need for examination

Remote consultations do not allow clinical examination and this should be considered carefully. Careful liaison with the referrer/general practitioner and appropriate triaging is key to organising these clinics.

Management problems

It is vital to ensure that the multidisciplinary team is aware of the comprehensive plan. Ensuring an adequate 'safety netting' provision is vital within the management plan. An individualised comprehensive management plan with adequate communication with the patient and general practitioner/referrer is key to a successful remote consultation.

Use of steroids during the COVID-19 pandemic

The Faculty of Pain Medicine released a statement on the use of steroids in pain procedures. They have issued a caution with regards to steroid use, as the immunological impact is not yet known. Risks should be clearly informed to patients if they are used. Pulsed radiofrequency and radiofrequency procedures can mitigate the use of steroids.

Key Points

- The difficult COVID-19 pandemic has forced us to change our working patterns in pain services.
- Remote consultations via telephone and web-based platforms have innovated pain service consultations.
- The use of steroids should be carefully considered and the risks should be explained to patients.

References

1. COVID-19: Guidance on triage and conducting quality consultations post COVID-19. Faculty of Pain Medicine of the Royal College of Anaesthetists, 2020. https://fpm.ac.uk/covid-19-guidance-triage-and-conducting-quality-consultations-post-covid-19. Accessed on 20th July 2020.

2. Pain practice post COVID-19. Triage — conducting quality consultations. Faculty of Pain Medicine of the Royal College of Anaesthetists, 2020. https://fpm.ac.uk/sites/fpm/files/documents/2020-06/Pain-Practice-Post-COVID-Triage-and-Consultations-June-2020.pdf. Accessed on 20th July 2020.

3. FPM response to concern related to the safety of steroids injected as part of pain procedures during the current COVID-19 virus pandemic. Faculty of Pain Medicine of the Royal College of Anaesthetists, 2020. https://fpm.ac.uk/sites/fpm/files/documents/2020-03/FPM-COVID-19-Steroid-Statement-2020-v2.pdf. Accessed on 20th July 2020.

Index

shingles 73, 74
     vaccine 76
sickle cell disease 95–101
sickle cell trait 95
Sievert (Sv) 170
SIGN guidelines 295
sleep disturbances 7, 184
SOCRATES 6–7, 26–7, 33–4
spinal cord stimulators 193–5, 293, 297
spinoreticular tract 17
spinothalamic tract 16
stellate ganglion block 147–51
steroids 281–4, 304
stochastic effects 171
structured assessment 6–12
stump pain 90, 91
substance misuse 201–5
surgical history 7
sympathetically mediated pain 45

T
tai-chi 177
talking therapies 185
tapentadol 241
TENS machines 176
tetracaine (amethocaine) 266, 267
     topical 274
third-order afferent fibres 17
Tinel's sign 91
topical agents 271–9
total pain 122
tramadol 240
transcutaneous electrical nerve stimulators (TENS) 176
transdermal drug delivery 275–6
transforaminal epidural 138, 139, 140
TransTec® patch 276
treatment history 7